Holistic Beauty from the Inside Out

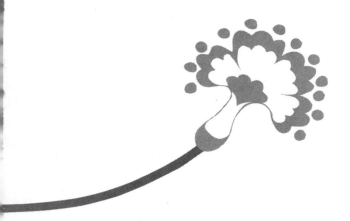

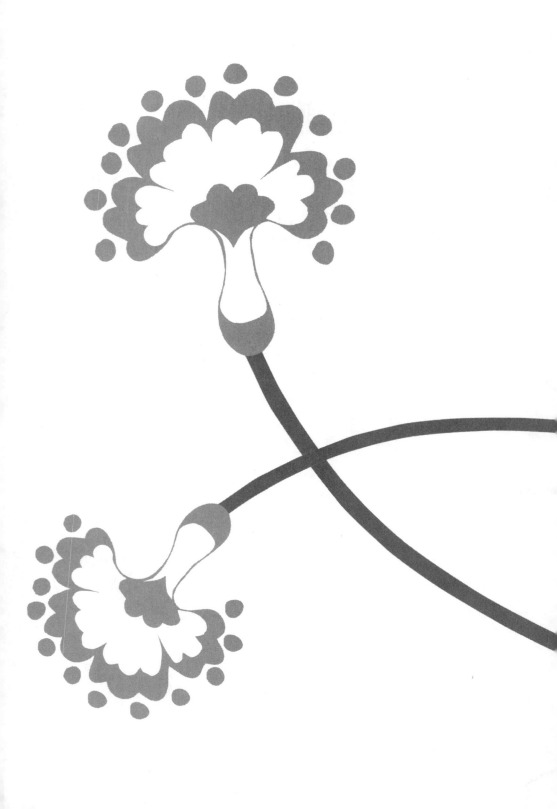

HOLISTIC BEAUTY
from the
INSIDE OUT

YOUR COMPLETE GUIDE
TO NATURAL HEALTH,
NUTRITION, AND
SKINCARE

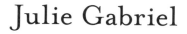

Julie Gabriel

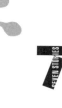

SEVEN STORIES PRESS
New York

SEVEN STORIES PRESS
140 Watts Street
New York, NY 10013
www.sevenstories.com

College professors may order examination copies of Seven Stories Press titles for a free six-month trial period. To order, visit http://www.sevenstories.com/textbook or send a fax on school letterhead to (212) 226-1411.

Library of Congress Cataloging-in-Publication Data
Gabriel, Julie.
Holistic beauty from the inside out : your complete guide to natural health, nutrition, and skincare / Julie Gabriel.— First edition.
    pages cm
ISBN 978-1-60980-461-9 (pbk.)
1. Women—Health and hygiene. 2. Holistic medicine. I. Title.
RA778.G228 2013
613'.04242—dc23
                              2012046140

Book design by Beth Kessler

Printed in the United States of America

9 8 7 6 5 4 3 2 1

I dedicate this book to the two lovely ladies in my life

Mama, you are so stunning,
I have no fear of growing older!

Maria, my lovely princess, you are so
naturally beautiful—please keep it that way!

CONTENTS

INTRODUCTION

In this modern world, is there a future for old-fashioned oatmeal scrubs, skin-firming masks with egg yolks and rye bread, and facial toners made of witch hazel and apple vinegar? In the age of the facelift, is there a place for meditation and stress-busting exercises? With all of the novel enzymes, nanoparticles, peptides, and vitamins at the disposal of today's dermatologist, shouldn't we all have glowing, youthful skin without a single blemish, wrinkle, or dark spot? Must our nightly slumber still be called "beauty sleep" if we can fix under-eye shadows with a magic gel? Do we still have to bother with herbs, clay, or oils in our bid to have gorgeous skin and lustrous hair?

Considering the astounding frequency of acne, eczema, dermatitis, hyperpigmentation, and hair loss we encounter today, it is clear that the cosmetic industry does not always deliver on its promises. Yet, somehow many of us still believe that all it takes to achieve glowing skin and lustrous hair is to slather on a potion that costs $20 a drop.

It is time to face the facts, ladies. During the last fifty years, the cosmetic industry has brainwashed women. We give away the responsibility for our own healthy appearance to cosmetics manufacturers who make fantastic claims that are rarely (if ever) based on human physiology—or plain ol' common sense. We are taught that we should rely on "magical" powers inside a glamorous jar or a futuristic-looking capsule, rather than on our bodies' own ability to preserve and improve our looks. If it's that expensive, we think, it surely must work! We seem to think that we have the same skin type, skin conditions, genetic makeup, metabolism, stress levels, and health concerns as thousands of other women who are buying the same jar, at the same minute, across the world. Even sports shoes come in a wider variety of options than skin cleansers in a regular department store.

Just as our brain is capable of producing the most powerful antidepressant known to science—namely, the neurotransmitter endorphin—our body is perfectly equipped with its own cleansing lotions, rejuvenating potions, and powerful skin-lifting serums to maintain and restore our natural beauty. Inside our bodies, we have enormous powers to rejuvenate our skin, hair, and nails without having to resort to expensive, often toxic, and sometimes even dangerous cosmetic procedures. Scrubs, masks, and laser treatments are nice and often beneficial, but even the most expensive cosmetic intervention cannot yield the lasting beauty we are after.

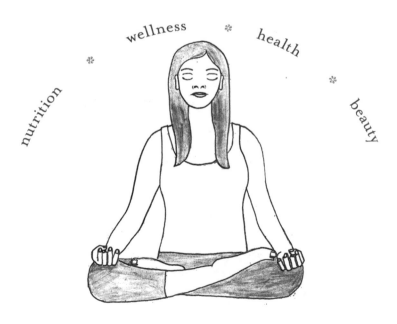

In this book you will discover how to take care of your skin, hair, and body in a holistic way, and come to understand why this approach makes more sense than addressing each issue with an isolated topical solution. You will learn about the healing powers of nutrition, sleep, and stress-relieving methods when it comes to skin, hair, nails, or perhaps any "wobbly bits" you may be concerned about.

For those with an interest in holistic health, you will find chapters that offer a "whole-body" approach to nutrition, wellness, health, and beauty. The advice is very practical and easy to follow. Just as it's not necessary to be a botanical expert to grow dill or parsley on your windowsill, similarly it's not necessary to be a nutritionist or a yoga expert to practice mindfulness, a beauty-boosting diet, and stress-relieving exercise. Most important, natural beauty should become the expression of your unique spirit and personality, which rules the way you treat your body and set up your mind.

As you read this book, you will learn how your skin absorbs nutritive and toxic substances, as well as what certain chemicals can do to your body and how to avoid the most dangerous ones. You will learn about the dangers of synthetic fragrances and parabens (preservatives), and you will understand why these cause allergies and increase your risk of heart disease, infertility, cancer, and other less invasive but still unpleasant health conditions. As soon as you realize that skincare products are food for your skin, you will be able to feed your skin right with "beauty meals." I am sure you know the health value of a homemade stew made with organic vegetables versus a hamburger with fries from a fast-food joint?

QUIT THE FAST FOOD BEAUTY HABIT

Beauty products have a lot in common with the foods that we eat. There are wholesome, nutrient-rich lotions and potions (and you can make a lot of them at home) and there are "fast-food" versions that you can find in any supermarket or pharmacy. These have little or no effect on overall health and well-being. At best, these blends of cheap petrochemicals and preservatives provide temporary relief from a specific discomfort. Maybe they make your skin feel less dry than usual. But the inner cause of dryness remains, so you reach for that plastic tube more and more often, and your skin itself makes no improvement.

When you understand the difference between "fast-food" and wholesome, natural beauty, you may decide to go a little longer on your way to a greener self. After you realize the premium you pay for packaging, storage, and transportation of conventional beauty products, not to mention their environmental impact, you will see the benefits of trying some easy recipes for organic, homemade skincare products. After you see how easy it is to make your own shampoo or body lotion, you will treat your skin and hair with more consideration and will shop for ready-made beauty products with more insight. You will become your own natural beauty expert. Add to that your newly gained knowledge of healing, beauty-promoting qualities of nutrition and stress relief, and nothing will stop you from becoming a true beauty, inside and out.

DETOX YOUR FACE

We all strive to look as best as we can. For some of us, money is not a restraint when it comes to the newest cosmetic procedure, or a scientific-seeming facial serum. For many others, it is an out-of-reach cure-all we regret not being able to afford. But what about health risks? Ninety percent of beauty products today are loaded with tongue-twisting chemical ingredients that promise instant results but have never been tested for long-term safety by reputable agencies. Even products labeled as "natural" and "organic" often contain synthetic additives that nearly nullify the benefits of botanicals and vitamins in the formula. Why should we risk our health in order to erase a wrinkle or fade a sun spot?

Choosing cosmetic ingredients that are effective yet harmless is not an easy task. Many antibacterial and antiseptic solutions, preservatives, alcohol, fragrances, silicones, and polymers used in conventional and natural skincare products may not be safe to use because of their allergenic and even carcinogenic potential. As the consumers, we have the right to know what is good and what is not working. Most often, if you cannot find a product that works for your skin condition, you can take the matter in your own hands and prepare the magic potion in your kitchen. It is very easy once you know how. Sometimes making your own skincare is the most economical solution. All beauty treatments and solutions in this book are entirely natural and chemical free.

This book contains product recommendations of natural and organic products that work really well for all skin and hair types. There are many excellent all-natural beauty products you can find in health food stores, natural groceries, pharmacies, and online, and I only recommend the ones that I have tested myself, with positive results.

When it comes to beauty, you have to become your own beauty expert, because no one else knows your skin, your diet, or your lifestyle better than you do. Your skin and hair conditions change every day. Your diet and your hormones can make or break that sleek, shiny hairstyle you have been anxious to achieve. So you need to be watchful, learn how to respond naturally to your skin and hair changes, and recognize when you need to be gentle or proactive, when you need to be a little more aggressive, or when you need to simply rest and wait. This book will empower you with the essential knowledge you need to make the decisions that are right for you. This book does not rely on folk wisdom and "magical" cures of yesteryears. Your skin is not the same as the skin your mother had twenty years ago. Water was different; air and food were less chemically loaded; skincare was less toxic.

We all are witnesses that creams alone cannot bring us youth, yet we all know that mere anticipation of a romantic date can tighten our skin better than any mask and brighten our eyes better than any eyedrops. An eight-hour sleep for a new mom can do wonders for her face. A meditation can diminish frowns and wrinkles. Falling in love can help us lose inches from our waistline, and brings that gorgeous glow to our cheeks that not a single bronzer can match.

In a real world, this amazing self-healing, self-beautifying capability of our bodies is undermined by the toxic environment we exist in. Contaminated water and air; synthetically enhanced, genetically modified, and processed food; artificial skincare; and pressures at work and home can wear out your looks, and age your skin and hair prematurely. This book explains why you should avoid parabens, aluminum, artificial fragrances and other estrogen mimickers as well as how they damage looks and health. Other environmental issues are raised, with a look at how slaughterhouse- and petroleum-derived ingredients in beauty products affect the environment. If you are unhappy with the current state of the unregulated beauty industry, its deceitful claims and self-admiring science, you will enjoy learning about self-reliant, inside-out beauty solutions that have very little negative impact on our amazing planet but have enormous positive effect on your health and state of mind.

HOLISTIC WAY OF BEAUTY

Are you one of those people who own a moisturizer for the face, a lotion for the oily T-zone, a cream for the eyes, another cream for the neck, a rich balm for the hands, and maybe three or five different masks that are diligently applied every night? Do you own separate creams for your feet, hands, bottom, and belly area? Do you treat your hair with at least five different products every morning, starting with shampoo, followed with a conditioner, straightener, volume-boosting foam, hair spray, and maybe a serum for split ends? Do you apply an antiperspirant topped with a spritz of a fragrance?

I bet you said yes to at least some of these questions. If you did, welcome to the world of synthetic beauty, where each and every skin area is treated in isolation from the rest of the body; where hair is simply a pretty accessory that needs to be dyed, glossed, ironed, and puffed; where nails are as glossy as your gel extensions permit; and where skin problems are managed with layers of expensive serums and acid peels, without real understanding of what's causing all those blemishes, spots, and wrinkles.

But there is another kind of beauty. It is called holistic beauty. The key word here is "holistic," a novel approach to beauty and well-being in general. Based on *holos*, a Greek word meaning "whole, entire," holistic health stresses that all aspects of our existence—psychological, physical, and social—should be taken into account and seen as a whole. Unlike symptomatic health, where symptoms are treated and not the whole body, holistic principles of well-being use natural diet, herbal remedies, nutritional supplements, relaxation, meditation, and alternative medicine practices such as acupuncture, homeopathy, and massage therapy to achieve the optimal state of well-being.

When it comes to beauty, holistic principles view our skin, hair, and nails not as visible body parts that need constant cleansing, polishing, painting, exfoliating, and dyeing to keep them pretty, but as integral parts of our well-being that can be improved with nutrition, relaxation, and probably a detox if exposed to synthetic toxins or suffering from congestion and possibly adverse conditions. Holistic beauty treats the face, body, hair, and nails as parts of the whole picture. Healthy skin and hair begin with the healthy liver, healthy bowels, healthy ovaries, and of course the healthy mind.

The holistic way of beauty teaches us to be proactive, not reactive. Instead of rubbing an expensive and potentially toxic cream into your wrinkles, let's try and prevent visible signs of aging with focused nutrition, supplements, sun protection, and stress relief. Instead of rubbing our skin with prescription medications to stop hair loss, turn to vitamins, acupuncture, and massage. Don't spend a fortune on gel nails if you can grow your own with simple changes in your diet and self-massage. Here is how holistic beauty interconnects all aspects of alternative medicine:

1. HEALTHY MIND. By adopting a positive mind-set, you will be less likely to make unhealthy choices in your diet or beauty regimen. When you stop falling prey to clever marketing and celebrity pressure, you will be able to fully concentrate on how your body feels and what you truly need to look and feel beautiful.

2. HEALTHY EMOTIONS. As you learn to stress less over minor things, you will enjoy a relaxed, glowing complexion with fewer blemishes and spots triggered by chronic stress. Nasolabial (nose to mouth) folds and forehead frowns will diminish, not because of expensive creams and injectable fillers, but thanks to relaxed facial muscles, improved circulation, and better sleep.

3. HEALTHY SKIN. When you stop being too demanding and anxious about your looks, clear skin and glowing hair follow. By eliminating unhealthy, toxic chemicals from your beauty routine and replacing them with natural alternatives, you are investing in the best health insurance possible—inside and out.

4. HEALTHY APPROACH. Equipped with knowledge about the healing powers of stress relief, healthy sleep, and natural skincare, you will become your own natural beauty expert who does not rely on store-bought kits and tools to deal with beauty dilemmas. Using simple natural ingredients and a little patience, you can deal with any cosmetic trouble, be it dry skin, blemishes, weak hair, brittle nails, or even cellulite.

ONE

Be Happy to Be Beautiful

There's no way around it: these days, we judge the book by its cover—and people by their looks. Of course we know that beauty is only skin deep, but we cannot ignore the simple fact: for better or worse, beauty matters. As defined by Webster's Dictionary, beauty can be summed up as "the qualities that give pleasure to the senses or exalt the mind." And we, humans, are all in for pleasure.

Beauty knows no time limits. A relief in the tomb of the Egyptian nobleman Ptahhotep, dating back to 2400 BC, shows the man getting a pedicure. Egyptians used milk and honey to cleanse their skin and made face masks of egg yolks and butter. Renaissance women plucked their hairline to achieve a desirable high forehead and lightened their hair with sulfur and onion hair dyes—they must have smelled as awful as our modern hair dyes do!

Beauty could be deadly. Renaissance women, who mastered the art of suffering in the name of beauty, rubbed their faces with whitening powders made of lead and mercury to achieve a fashionable white pallor. Victorian women constricted their ribs in quest for thinner waistline and swallowed worms to obtain translucent skin. These days, women happily sacrifice their comfort for beauty every time they struggle into a pair of Spanx, or pluck unwanted hairs, one by one, from their eyebrows. How different is the ancient Chinese custom of foot binding from modern-day six-inch heels towering over three-inch platforms? Or Victorian rib-sawing from today's unchallenged custom of filling the breasts with petrochemicals through the daily use of toxic products?

Beauty is money, and a lot of it. In the United States in 2011, people spent $6 billion on fragrance and another $6 billion on makeup.[1] Hair- and skincare products drew $8 billion each, while nail products accounted for $1 billion. In the United States alone, $20 billion are spent each year on diet, weight-loss products, and club memberships, while $10 billion go toward cosmetic surgery bills, despite record unemployment, mounting health care costs, and plummeting home values.

Beauty discriminates. Studies suggest that attractive people make more money, receive lighter court sentences, and are perceived as friendlier and more desirable partners. Clear skin, glossy hair, clear eyes, and a slender body announce, "I'm healthy and fertile. I make a welcome addition to the gene pool." They increase the woman's pool of romantic partners and widen the range of opportunities in her work and day-to-day life.

"Beautiful people get all the breaks," says psychologist Victoria Fleming, author of *You Complete Me and Other Myths that Destroy Happily Ever After.* "Our society teaches us to be obsessed with looks. But on a more basic level, our looks are what draw that first impression someone has about us. First impressions are based on visual judgments. The brain does this automatically. And frankly, technology today puts the pressure up even higher because there's not a lot of rebound time if your first impression isn't good! One click and you are literally off the radar."

Smooth skin, big eyes, curvaceous bodies, and full lips serve as reliable signals of youth, good health, and fertility. Psychologists found that men have instinctive penchant for women with large eyes, full lips, and a small nose and chin, while women prefer men who are taller than they are with symmetrical features. Recent studies also show that men have an instinctive preference for the classic hourglass-shaped body with a waist-hip ratio of 7:10.[2] The state of the skin is an important signal too. Millennia of evolution make us instinctively suspect infections, parasites, and general poor health in people whose skin is plagued by lesions and spots. On the contrary, clear, glowing skin equals health and well-being.[3]

WOULD YOU EAT A PLASTIC BAG?

We have all got bits of ourselves we are not particularly thrilled with. Let's be honest: I don't like my tummy, and for very good reason. It's flabby and bumpy, and no amount of crunches seem to make any difference. But here's the question: Do I despise my tummy or the way my tummy *looks*? Covered in cellulite or not, the inner workings of my tummy—such as stomach, liver, bowels, kidneys, uterus, ovaries—function just fine, and I have no reason to dislike them. It's the skin texture and the profile in the mirror that I don't like.

Same with legs, hair, or ears. Many women dislike their legs and wish they were longer, thinner, or with less cellulite. But what about the daily work our legs do for us? What about places they take us to, steps they march up or down, sometimes in shoes that are clearly not fit for walking? Still hate your hair and think it makes you look less pretty? Then think how you'd look if you lost all of your hair after cancer treatment. You would be thankful to be alive, that is. Hair, or the lack thereof, would become a lesser concern.

Most of us hate our bodies for no good reason—until our bodies are being taken from us because of illness or other circumstances. According to sad statistics, only 3 percent of women with an average age of thirty-three are happy with their body, while six out of ten women say their body makes them feel depressed. A total of 91 percent of women were unhappy with their hips and thighs, 77 percent with their waist, and 78 percent complained of cellulite.[4] That's when we reach for a lip liner, a new cellulite serum, or make an appointment with a hair stylist or a dermatologist.

"There are at least two parts to a woman's self-concept—how she feels about herself on the inside, and how she feels about herself on the outside," says Dr. Fleming. "What's on the inside might be an uncontrollable mess. She feels insecure. She feels unloved. She feels unworthy. And these may be deep-seated feelings that she feels powerless to change! What's on the outside she has a little more control over. She can fix her makeup to look just right. She can use the same perfume as Taylor Swift. Or she can just take on the latest trends as part of her identity, so that she fits in where otherwise she feels like an outsider. It distracts them from 'ugly' truths they want to avoid. It gives them a sense of control. Trying to help women understand that true beauty comes from within is a tough sell, because of all the reinforcement they get—and see others getting—for the physical beauty."

The celebrity-driven beauty industry plants unrealistic images into our minds, and, in order to achieve the looks from the magazine pages or a TV screen, we are prompted to dye, straighten, erase, elongate, straighten, lift, polish, blow-dry, buy, buy, buy, and then buy some more. Not all of these efforts are for pure vanity's sake. In their quest for longer lashes or smoother skin, women are really seeking love, acceptance, and success. "Sometimes that fastest route to that goal is to align themselves with others who are clearly loved, accepted, and successful—a.k.a., the celebrity," notes Dr. Fleming, "There is a term called *BIRGing*— Basking in Reflected Glory. I may not get the glory myself, but if I stand close enough to you, some of that light will bounce over to me. When the celebrities are out of the spotlight, they have the same doubts and esteem issues as everyone else, but they put the best of themselves out there for public consumption, and women eat it up."

The gap between the cultural stereotypes of what we are expected to look like and the reality of what we actually look like is becoming wider than ever before. In one of its worst manifestations, discontent with one's body can devolve into an eating disorder or obsession with plastic surgery. In less extreme cases, some women feel obliged to spend up to half their monthly income on creams, gels, serums, and lotions.

Dr. Fleming explains that pampering can be quite healthy expression of self-care: I love myself; therefore, I take care of myself. "It's not necessarily a bad thing to indulge in caring for the self, particularly for women who are missing a sense of love and safety from a partner or from their family. If you grow up being told you are not worthy and don't deserve nice things, then indulging yourself with creams and lotions could be a healthy defiance of those negative messages. Some of the best cosmetic tag lines over the years reinforce healthy esteem—"'Because I'm worth it,'" comes to mind immediately. But the issue is that it's gone too far. Women are using beauty products as a replacement for healthy esteem and self-love, rather than as an expression of it. I think that's where the trouble starts."

That's when the "hope in a jar" takes root. Fresh-faced teenage girls advertising wrinkle creams only add to the confusion. The only true hope that exists in a jar belongs to the CEO selling it. He hopes that you (and millions of others) will have enough hope to buy him a new jet, a new boat, and a new villa in France.

At any moment, in any cosmetic department in any shopping mall, there are a growing number of women who don't feel like being duped. They have a healthy, realistic relationship with beauty accepting it as the ticket to better relationships, increased career opportunities, and generally more rewarding life. As they age, they simply take pride in their wrinkles and silver hair, trying to look like sensual, older women, not like fifty going on twenty.

The healthy approach to beauty is neither pretending it's shallow or unnecessary, nor being preoccupied with it. Being honest about your personal value of beauty helps you make informed decisions on how much effort, time, and money to spend on your appearance.

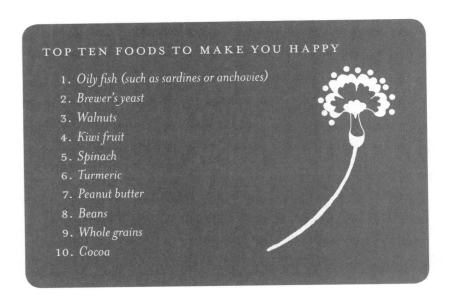

TOP TEN FOODS TO MAKE YOU HAPPY

1. *Oily fish (such as sardines or anchovies)*
2. *Brewer's yeast*
3. *Walnuts*
4. *Kiwi fruit*
5. *Spinach*
6. *Turmeric*
7. *Peanut butter*
8. *Beans*
9. *Whole grains*
10. *Cocoa*

THE INNER SENSE OF BEAUTY

"At the core of every human being is a profound need to have value," says Dr. Fleming. "The more a person is convinced of their self-worth, the less they need validation from other sources. There is a difference in what women and men need for validation. With a man, his self-esteem is stronger when he is respected and appreciated. With a woman, her self-esteem is strengthened when she is given attention and valued. Parents who provide these to their children consistently from an early age have children who become rock-solid in their inner security."

I am not here to lecture on parenting, but for many of us,

something went seriously wrong at one point in our childhood or teenage years. For how else can you explain that when it comes to body image, women are champions of self-depreciation and gurus of self-punishment? If you flick through the typical women's magazine, all of the women therein must be tall and flat-stomached, with shiny, perfectly white teeth, and laugh like mad while devouring a plateful of salad (Do they eat some special kind of salad on those photo shoots?). And here you look in the mirror, making a mental note of your blemishes, wrinkles, and double chin, and realize you just aren't beautiful and therefore you are not desirable or successful. How does that make you feel?

We all want to look good—and I know you do too, otherwise you wouldn't be reading this book. We could all throw up our arms and surrender completely to Mother Nature, go totally au naturel and say, "Hair coloring is for sissies!" But most of us want to look good, smell good, radiate health, and manage what we were born with in a way that makes the most of ourselves, without it turning into a battle of hatred. So, how do you find a balance between accepting yourself and still caring about how you look? Here are some ideas how to learn to feel good in the skin you are in.

REDEFINE "BEAUTY"

You eat a balanced diet, you fit activity into your daily routine, and you enjoy yourself when you're out with friends rather than fret over how many calories you're consuming. Isn't that healthier than being at a certain weight or size? Beauty is about feeling great about yourself, and if you're killing yourself trying to look "pretty"—for example, baking in a tanning salon, inhaling formaldehyde fumes during a weekly hair straightening session, or inject toxins to smooth out wrinkles—something is wrong with your approach.

"There was a saying a few years ago that went, 'Love the skin you're in.' I think the way out of the rut is to turn your attention from the external to the internal," says psychologist Dr. Fleming.

"You are a spiritual being having an earthly experience. That internal light, that spirit, is the most important part of who you are. There is research that has looked at 'Quality of Life' measures among people dying from cancer. They expected quality of life to decline, but they hadn't counted on people finding new value in spirit while their bodies declined. It revealed that very often it isn't until the body is in decline that people get that they are more than this physical form. Their spirit has little to do with the container!"

FOCUS ON "NOW"

Too many people spend too much time regretting the past or fearing the future. Beauty-wise, regretting all the silly things we did to our skin and hair, having too much sun, too much smoking, or alcohol leads to fretting the future with all its wrinkles, sagging, liver spots, and gray hair, not to mention other age-related health issues. This "mental diet" of regret and fear will age your skin and hair quicker than you think. Every minute you waste disliking a part of yourself is a minute less of your life. When you're eighty-five years old and look back, will you be glad that you spent so much time worrying about your skin and hair? If you get caught in the regret/fear circle too often, simply bring attention to this very moment and try to catch that moment of peace and serenity that feels like *now*.

THINK "PRETTY" THOUGHTS

Remember that we can make our own thoughts. No one thinks in the same way, and making other people think like us is a waste of precious mental energy. It's your thoughts, not life's challenges, that make you truly positive and happy about yourself. Only you, not the outside world, can dictate how you feel. Throw out all the "mental junk food" that overwhelms your brain. Negative thought patterns varying from "I am so fat, I will never meet someone," to "I am so old and ugly," should go down the drain so that you could fill your mental space with wholesome, positive thinking patterns that make you feel and look better. Healthy thoughts will make your skin glow and eyes sparkle.

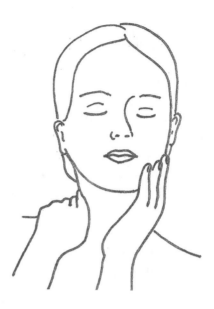

A great example of this technique that is easy to incorporate into your life is the use of positive affirmations. Pick a few positive and validating phrases, and repeat them to yourself throughout the day. "I am beautiful" is a wonderful and simple affirmation. Simply repeat the phrase to yourself, either aloud or in your head, and imagine yourself at your most beautiful. Do this while cooking dinner, driving to work, doing the laundry, brushing your teeth—whenever your mind is likely to roam. Eventually, you will notice that this positive, life-affirming phrase will start to pop up into your head all on its own, and replace some of the old negative self-talk. Filling your mind with positive affirmations has the power to change your whole attitude, and imbue you with a confidence and appreciation for life that is often accompanied by a gorgeous, energetic glow.

STOP CRITICIZING

A critical state of mind bites other people and eats you alive. Some people get an instant "high" from wagging their acrid tongues, but in fact criticizing others is a quick but dishonest way to praise yourself. In the long run, all this negativity spilled at others damages your own self-esteem. If we cannot achieve certain things that we have always wanted, then we begin complaining and criticizing others. When you feel comfortable in your own skin, you are not threatened or offended by the imperfections you see in others. Being less critical and judgmental of other people makes you kinder and more accepting of your own flaws and imperfections that make you unique. When you encounter new acquaintances, make it a goal to look for something you like about them, and pay them a compliment. As you go through you day with your loved ones and coworkers, do the same for them. When you seek out the beauty and admirable features in those around you, you will find yourself in an ever-increasingly beautiful universe.

Being less critical can extend beyond those around you, to your general view on life. Keeping a gratefulness journal is an excellent daily practice that has transformative effects, and takes merely one or two minutes a day. Simply write down what you are most grateful for each night in a journal that you keep in your bedroom. It could be a gorgeous full moon, a particularly delicious piece of fruit, or your baby's first word. Whatever you choose each night, the practice of searching for what you are most grateful for helps you to put on some rose-colored glasses that will help you to encounter, and therefore experience, the world less critically. After this becomes habit, you will find yourself looking for things to be grateful for throughout the day, and finding lots of beautiful possibilities you may never have noticed before.

DECIDE WHAT'S BEST FOR YOU

All of us make decisions on a daily basis. "Life is the sum of all your choices," wrote Albert Camus. When it comes to your looks, your main goal is to be comfortable with your decisions. Heavy makeup and elaborate hair styles make you annoyingly aware of your body all day, stripping away your confidence and filling you up with negativity which can ruin all the efforts you make to prettify yourself. If a no-makeup face and no-hairspray hair make you feel good in your skin, do so rather than try to squeeze yourself into the image you think is trendy and "fashionable" right now.

PRAISE YOURSELF

A common thought for many women is, "If I have blotchy skin, if I have dull hair, if my thighs are wobbly, if I'm not thin enough, no one will want me." That's a terrible mind-set that can lead to sheer obsession with appearance. If you heard these statements from someone else, you would call them hurtful. Yet, we allow us to hurt ourselves all the time. Next time when you take a critical look in the mirror, think about the amazing machine your body is. Your eyes can read and cry, no matter what size and color they are. Your legs can run and bike, even if you forget to wax them. Your tummy can grow little people inside of you—yes, even when covered with cellulite. How amazing! Instead of criticizing what your body *looks like*, show it a little love by appreciating what it *does*. How often do you focus who you are as a person instead of how you look? Do you ever say, "Good job, my sweetheart!" or even pat yourself on the shoulder? Hug yourself and even dot a little kiss at your hand for being positive and kind to yourself. Self-compassion and self-acceptance are the cornerstones of healthy attitude toward beauty. Continual judgment and criticism of our looks keeps us locked in a continuous cycle of unhappiness with our looks, our faces, and ultimately our lives.

IMAGINE YOURSELF BEAUTIFUL

You can take charge of your thoughts and guide your imagination toward a relaxed, focused state where you see yourself as an attractive, confident person with glowing skin and a slender, healthy body. Guided imagery is a program of directed thoughts and suggestions that involve all of your senses.

Here's a simple exercise that demonstrates the immense power of imagination over our well-being. Visualize a lemon in slightest detail: its yellow dotty skin, the shiny surface, the oval shape, the pungent smell. Continue to imagine the taste of the lemon and then imagine yourself taking a bite of the fruit. Feel the tangy juice squirting into your mouth. Do you salivate? I bet you do. Now you can see how eagerly our body responds to what you are imagining.

You can use guided imagery technique to achieve a relaxed state of mind and improve your self-acceptance, health, and sense of well-being. Imagine a safe, comfortable place, such as a beach or a garden, in a great detail. Lie comfortably on the floor or recline on a sofa.

Take a few slow, even breaths. When you are feeling relaxed, gently close your eyes. Picture yourself lying on a beautiful secluded beach or a lovely garden full of flowers. Picture soft white sand around you, or maybe soft grass caressing your body. Imagine a cloudless sky above and green leaves gently moving in the warm breeze. Feel the warm touch of mellow sun on your skin. Enjoy the sound of the waves gently rolling onto shore or birds chirping in the trees around you.

Breathe in and smell the scent of the ocean and the aroma of flowers. Picture yourself looking young, with glowing skin and glossy hair, dressed in a beautiful and comfortable outfit.

Stay in this scene for as long as you like. Notice how relaxed and calm you feel. Notice how the tension melts throughout your entire body, from your head to your toes. Notice how insignificant your worries and fears look when you have surrounded yourself with peace and quiet.

When the time is up (start with fifteen minutes twice a day), slowly count backward from ten. Open your eyes.

During guided imagery, our body seems to respond as though what you are imagining is real. When you imagine yourself free from stresses and looking naturally gorgeous, our body follows the "command."

BOOST YOUR HAPPINESS HORMONE

They say that life is like a zebra: a black stripe will inevitably end, and the white stripe will begin. But sometimes it seems that we wander endlessly *along* the black stripe, not crossways. That's when the nature's most powerful antidepressant comes handy—and to try it, you don't need a prescription, and the side effects are only positive.

This antidepressant is called endorphins. It's actually a group of opioids created naturally in the body. The word "endorphin" itself is built from two words: *endogenous morphins*—that is, narcotic substances produced naturally in the body. Like morphine, endorphins raise the pain threshold and produce sedation and euphoria. Endorphins are responsible for so-called "runner's high," which helps athletes push themselves beyond their physical and mental limits, feeling no exhaustion or pain. Endorphins are released during pregnancy, which partially explains post-partum depression as the mother is deprived of endorphins in her system and the nerve-soothing effect of breastfeeding when endorphins are released into her blood. What a timely gift of nature, considering all those sleepless nights and physical and emotional exhaustion during the day!

To achieve a true endorphin kick, you don't need to exhaust yourself with running spurts. In fact, moderate exercise followed by a relaxation technique—for example, a massage or meditation—also triggers the release of endorphins. Basically, all prolonged rhythmic exercises, such as tennis and aerobics, boost the production of body's own "happiness hormone." Meditation, acupuncture, deep diaphragm breathing, even eating spicy food—all these simple steps help maintain steady levels of this feel-good chemical in the blood. Certain foods also come in handy, especially stimulating foods such as chili peppers, horseradish, and wasabi.

No wonder exercise is increasingly becoming a part of the treatment of depression and anxiety. Regular physical activity appears as effective as psychotherapy for treating mild to moderate depression.[5] Chinese therapists also report that patients who exercise regularly, especially practicing mind-body exercise such as tai chi, are less likely to experience cognitive decline in old age.[6]

> *For a smooth transition from a couch potato to a running beauty, enjoy Wii Fit activities such as yoga, muscle conditioning, balance, and aerobics and develop a taste for more vigorous, real-life exercise.*

It appears that nearly any form of exercise can help boost your mood with endorphin release. Some examples of happiness-boosting exercise include:

- Biking or spinning class
- Nordic walking or uphill walking
- Dancing
- Golf (but only if you walk instead of using the cart)
- Jogging
- Aerobics
- Kickboxing or martial arts
- Tennis
- Swimming
- Yoga

Gardening, yard work (especially mowing or raking), and housework (such as sweeping, mopping, or vacuuming) also count as endorphin-boosting exercises. At least I know now what prompts me to grab a broom when I feel low and the sky is overcast!

Before you begin an exercise program for mood boost, you may ask yourself if there are any particular physical activities you enjoy or if they fit your lifestyle and work schedule. Some people enjoy working out in a club atmosphere while others opt for lonely runs in the wilderness. Choose an activity you enjoy. Exercising should be fun, otherwise you will not continue.

You also need to be clear about your goals. When you first start your exercise program, it should be easy for you to follow and maintain. For example, if you aim for mood enhancement, then weight loss and improved flexibility will inevitably follow after you begin your workouts in your spare time. But if you are after strong, voluptuous muscles, you will need to be prepared to spend at least an hour every day in the gym. Put your exercise routine into your schedule.

Variety is the key to enjoying life at its fullest. Choose at least three activities from the list above and try to incorporate them into your monthly exercise schedule. Most often, you don't need to buy health club memberships or expensive equipment to enjoy endorphin-boosting activities. All you need to run is a pair of trainers and a flat surface. All you need to do crunches is a flat surface.

When you have made up your mind to fit some fitness into your life, keep the timer on. It takes about thirty minutes between the start of an exercise and a full release of endorphins, so make sure you time your fitness routine just right. Here are is a simple exercise sequence to boost your happiness naturally with endorphins:

1. TREADMILL: Start with a five-minute warm up at a comfortable speed. Then, every three minutes, increase both the speed and difficulty. Incline the treadmill one increment and increase speed. On a bike, increase the resistance and maintain the same cadence. Do this four times, so that you can exercise for twelve to fifteen minutes with ever-increasing intensity.

2. CRUNCHES: The essential move to get your tummy into tip-top shape for bikini season, it's also one of the most reliable endorphin triggers—although I

get a secondary happiness boost when I notice less flabbiness around the waist area! Crunches are tricky, so do them right. Here's the simplest way to do crunches without hurting your back:

- Lie on your back with your knees bent and feet flat on the ground.
- Place your hands behind your head with your elbows out and arms horizontal. Do not bend your arms forward.
- Supporting your head with your hands, squeeze your abs until your upper torso is just off the floor. Pause for one second.
- Slowly release your abs and roll back your spine to the starting position. Do not pull your hands onto your neck.
- As your core muscles become stronger, you can start working your lower abs, completing a crunch with your body bent at a 90-degree angle at the hips, and your legs shooting straight up in the air.
- For optimum endorphin release (and a flatter tummy), complete three sets, twenty repetitions each. Start with ten reps and work your way to twenty.

3. WEIGHT LIFTING: You do not need to move a lot of iron to see endorphins in action and your muscles gaining firmness and definition. Spend ten to fifteen minutes waving some dumbbells around (ten to fifteen repetitions for arm muscles). If you are not in the mood for spending lots of money on sports equipment, fill up two textured 1.5 L (1.59 qt) plastic bottles with water and use them as weights on a treadmill. You can add weight to your makeshift dumbbells by stuffing some sand or gravel into the bottles, along with water.

After your endorphin-boosting workout, you will feel a mild sense of euphoria and walk through your day with a greater spring in your step. You will likely sleep better that night too.

ENHANCE YOUR RELATIONSHIPS

Keep up your connections with your loved ones and close friends, and make sure that you don't de-prioritize them in the face of ever-mounting deadlines and pressures at work and in life. Schedule automatic weekly or monthly lunch dates with friends who make you feel good and rejuvenate you. Plan Skype or phone appointments with family and friends who are too far away to see regularly. Spend quality time with your family, without the television in the room! Make time every day to play a board game, go outside for a walk, or dance around the house to your favorite music with your nearest and dearest. These are the moments of life that feed the soul.

DO WHAT YOU LOVE

This one seems simple, but it seems to be the first thing that gets thrown off the to-do list in our busy lives. Do something creative that you enjoy every day. Have you always wanted to write a novel or play the guitar? Do you enjoy knitting or scrapbooking? Commit yourself to engaging in this activity for just ten minutes every day. Everyone can commit to ten minutes, even if you do it just before going to sleep, just after waking up, while waiting for the dryer to finish a load, or during a quick break at work. If you feel inspired, or find yourself with more time, go onward. But, make sure that you meet your ten minutes, even in the busy times. Life is meant to be lived passionately, and those ten minutes just might fill you with the vigor you've been missing!

If all else fails, and you are not happy and you know it, consider adopting a pet. Pets can provide a lot of positive psychological and physical benefits for their owners. First of all, pets themselves are a great social support, and they can help you to meet fellow humans who can provide social support as well. Dog owners socialize at canine playgrounds; lizard owners have their fun too, undoubtedly.

Scientific studies have found that pet owners enjoy increased well-being, such as greater self-esteem, greater conscientiousness, less fearful attachment, and more exercise. Pets are unconditionally supportive, and their ability to improve their owners' self-esteem is beyond any comparison. But perhaps most important, pets are actually able to stave off negativity caused by social rejection.[7]

Chapter One Quick Tips

1. **Don't sacrifice your long-term health** for a minute of a joy when you look at your newly puffy lips, newly smooth skin, or temporarily wrinkle-free forehead. A reflection in the mirror is gone within seconds, but the poison inside of you may take months to take its toll.

2. **Be kind to yourself.** Love your legs, arms, eyes, and ears, as well as the rest of your body. You do not criticize the way people's children look (I hope!). Then why be critical about the way your *own* body looks? Our life throws tons of outside critics our way; let's become our body's major supporter. Give your inner critic a *hard* boot. Remember: happy people live longer.

3. **Be thankful.** Women are champions of unhappiness and dissatisfaction with their looks. A bad day at work, problems within a relationship, or even a misdirected word can lead to grumpy feelings about your nose, thighs, or belly. Say "thank you" to your body for serving you so faithfully. No matter what your physical or mental condition, things almost certainly could be worse. Cultivate a sense of appreciation for any of the five senses that still operate effectively: taste, touch, sight, sound, and smell. The smell of a perfume, the sight of a flower, the crunch of freshly baked bread, the touch of a snowflake, and the taste of an excellent cup of coffee can bring a smile to anyone's face, so enjoy these pleasures while you can. You don't need pouty lips or shimmery blond hair to enjoy life at its fullest.

4. **Get rid of mental junk food** such as thoughts that were processed beyond recognition. Do not plaster yourself with truisms and negative thought patterns. They only clutter your mind and never give you anything good in return. Try eliminating all the junk and focusing on positive, wholesome thoughts, and kind acts toward yourself. Nourish your soul with positive "food" in forms of positive thinking, meditation, and relaxation, and your skin and hair will follow the lead toward a prettier future.

5. **Nurture your mind with positive experiences** rather than rewarding buys. Every day devote at least ten minutes to something you love, be it reading, painting, jumping on a trampoline, cycling, or gardening. By ditching junk habits such as spending a night in front of a television, you will find more than enough time to spend with your loved ones—including one-on-one time with another person you should love—yourself.

TWO

Relax to Be Beautiful

Many of us are working long hours, juggling careers with family life, struggling in a bad economy, and waking up before the sun rises to hide our fears and worries under a heavy concealer, a blow-dry, and some shimmering blush. No wonder many of us are surviving on a steady supply of caffeine, nicotine, and adrenaline, and remain barely able to cope. Unfortunately, we often allow such stresses to accompany us for years.

We now know that living with chronic stress has serious consequences for our health and well-being, contributing to everything from bad moods to heart disease. Stress has become the main cause of long-term sickness and absence from work, overtaking acute illnesses such as cancer.[8] Stress is also the number one enemy of your beauty. The damage begins in our brain, when chronic stress causes the hypothalamus, a tiny gland often called by doctors as the "brain's brain," to decline in function. As the hypothalamus declines, it triggers dysfunction of the rest of the endocrine system, which causes damage to the body and the mind.

Immunity declines. Fat accumulates around the waistline. Eye muscles lose their tone. Skin loses elasticity and flexibility, and hair starts falling out.

Aside from its direct destructive effect on our immune and endocrine systems, chronic stress creates a new set of beauty-related worries for us. If you have a tendency toward acne, stress will keep those nasty blemishes popping up, despite all your efforts to keep your skin clear.

As if undermining our healthy looks were not enough, stress makes us its ally in its war against beauty. When we are stressed out and anxious, we make poor choices that directly affect the condition of our skin and hair. We replace water with tea and coffee setting up for puffiness, dry skin, and dark eye circles. We reach for the glass of wine or a cigarette, load up on "comfort" foods which are usually fatty, sweet, and filled to the brim with empty calories. How do we stop worrying and learn to be beautiful?

STRESS HORMONES SPEED UP AGING

When we live with chronic stress, our skin is the first to suffer. Some people living under constant pressure can develop hives (urticaria), itch (pruritus), skin flushing, and sweating, even hair loss (alopecia). Chronic stress can also lead to acne, psoriasis, eczema, and premature skin aging.

When you suffer from chronic stress, your adrenal glands (two small triangular glands that sit atop of the kidneys) become overworked. Adrenals produce vital stress-regulating hormones, mainly cortisol and adrenaline. In a situation of a psychological stress, the increased levels of cortisol inhibit the release of free radical scavenging enzyme called superoxide dismutase.[9] This weakens your body's natural defenses and leaves your skin vulnerable to environmental pollutants. In fact, chronic stress is one of the chief contributors to an increased population of free radicals in your body, which causes premature aging. Low levels of superoxide lead to chronic inflammation that brings a host of visible skin problems including acne, eczema, rashes, and early wrinkles.

Stress also depletes your skin of oxygen. As the kidneys produce more adrenaline, blood is directed away from your skin and is sent to your muscles to deal with emergency situations. Your skin receives fewer nutrients and oxygen resulting in a dull, pale, sallow complexion.

Stress also undermines digestion. Now, your body cannot absorb all the nutrients from the foods you eat while undigested impurities accumulate faster than your body can get rid of them. Dead skin cells take longer to turn over, skin cell production is diminished, and collagen and elastin production slows. Result? Dark eye circles and eye puffiness, blemishes, sagging skin, dilated pores, and rough, uneven skin texture. That's hardly a pretty picture.

As if that weren't enough, muscles tend to get stiff and tense as a reaction to stress. Aside from slowing down the circulation in the skin, stiff facial muscles form folds and creases, which deepen with time. Have you ever noticed how smooth and calm your face becomes during a vacation when you are less exposed to the mental toxins of daily life?

NUTRITIOUS NIRVANA

Diet and exercise are the most powerful and completely natural means to diminish our daily stress load. Our brains and nervous systems do not function well on a steady influx of fast food, sugar, white flour, and processed meat. They need real nourishment.

Of all the diets that are helpful to relieve stress, the Mediterranean diet is best. A recent study found that a typical Mediterranean diet reduces the risk of depression by nearly one third. Spanish researchers found that people who regularly eat a lot of vegetables, fruits, nuts, and oily fish are 30 percent less likely to suffer from anxiety and depression than those whose diet is not a Med-style.[10] This type of a diet also calls for reduced consumption of meats and whole-fat dairy. Scientists from the University of Navarra found that the Mediterranean diet, with its high content of essential fatty acids from fish and olive oil plus antioxidants and bio-available vitamins in fresh produce, reduces inflammatory and metabolic processes that trigger depression.[11] Chapter Four of this book will provide a detailed look at what a healthy, stress-busting diet might look like. However, it is important to note a couple things about *how* you eat here, as it relates to stress.

What, how, and when we eat also affects our brain chemistry. "The wrong foods can affect our moods and emotions. On the flip side, our emotions can affect our gut health which then is reflected on our skin," says yoga teacher Devinder Kaur. "If we experience a lot of fear, especially fear of criticism, we end up creating tension in our gut, which then affects our ability to eliminate. When there is chronic constipation, our skin, which mirrors our gut, will reflect this problem." Staying regular by eating slowly and consciously while sitting down, including lots of fiber in your diet, and drinking lots of water is therefore a big part of health!

Missing a meal can turn some people into monsters. Luckily, the best foods for positive thinking also help rejuvenate your skin and hair. Think oily fish, whole grains, cheese, avocado, nuts, and all the fruits and vegetables you fancy. To avoid a midday slump and maintain a positive mood, don't skip meals so that your blood sugar levels remain even. Pair proteins with minimally processed whole grains—this will supply your body with slow-releasing carbohydrates that will keep your blood sugar levels stable. If your moods falls below zero, keep your mind clear with a fruit rather than sweets or coffee.

To keep your emotions in balance, our brain needs B vitamins and magnesium from unrefined grains such as brown rice, wheat germ, and nuts and seeds (especially almonds, walnuts, and sunflower seeds). If you eat meat, that's a good source of B vitamins too, but choose organic and free-range meats to minimize your exposure to toxic chemicals found in conventionally produced meat.

Vitamins of the B group are perhaps the most reliable stress busters in the vitamin realm. They support mechanisms that help our bodies cope with physical and mental stress, promote better body chemistry, and even restore vital neurotransmitter functions. For example, vitamin B3 (niacin) works for fatigue, anxiety, and even depression—but only in large doses. Still, if you take only 100 mg daily (best if you consult with your medical practitioner, just to be sure), you will notice positive effects such as clear thinking and better control of your emotions. Another B vitamin, pyridoxine (B6), is simply a godsend to women who suffer from premenstrual syndrome (PMS) and water retention before their periods.

Minerals needed to promote stress relief include zinc, magnesium, potassium, and manganese. Low zinc levels have been associated with low mood and unstable emotions. Magnesium is often called a "mineral antidepressant" and is best taken at bedtime. Manganese, ideally taken as a part of a well-formulated multivitamin from a reputable brand, helps the synthesis of dopamine, a mood-balancing neurotransmitter that also helps calm down and soothe the nerves.

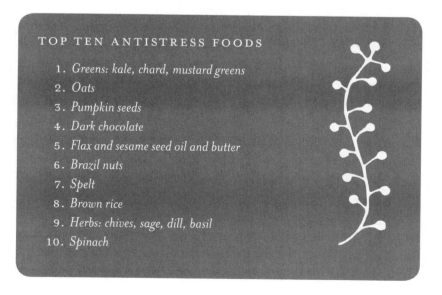

TOP TEN ANTISTRESS FOODS

1. *Greens: kale, chard, mustard greens*
2. *Oats*
3. *Pumpkin seeds*
4. *Dark chocolate*
5. *Flax and sesame seed oil and butter*
6. *Brazil nuts*
7. *Spelt*
8. *Brown rice*
9. *Herbs: chives, sage, dill, basil*
10. *Spinach*

Another great stress-reducer is garlic. It is especially useful if you think that your anxiety or jittery mood is due to sugar cravings, or ups and downs in your blood sugar levels. Garlic acts as a mop for substances that deactivate insulin, so that you enjoy increased available insulin and, as a result, more stable blood sugar levels. In people with diabetes, garlic improves blood sugar regulation and energy balance, but if you do not have diabetes, you can also put these amazing qualities of garlic to your own health use. You can make garlic bread (make sure to use whole wheat loaves), or add some fresh garlic to your pasta sauce (by the way, tomato in your pasta is a powerful scavenger of free radicals and can even help protect from sunburn and premature aging). Asian stir-fries also call for large quantities of garlic. You can take garlic as an infused oil in capsules—this is perhaps the least smelly way to add more garlic phytochemicals to your diet.

With proper use, herbs can be a godsend when we are at our most tense and harried. By calming down your nerves, antistress herbs slow down the release of stress hormones, which, in turn, diminishes the chronic inflammation and normalizes skin functions, so it's not dry, itchy, or flaking anymore.

To achieve a Zen state of peace and calm, some of us need a natural boost, and some need a natural soother. When it comes to calming your nerves, the sweet-smelling chamomile (*Matricaria recutita*) is extremely helpful. Chamomile can be a miraculous mood balancer for young and old—it can even be used on newborn babies suffering from colic and digestive problems. The best way to enjoy chamomile is to sip a golden-hued herbal tea prepared with whole flowers or tea bags. You can also add chamomile to your bath for whole body relaxation.

Valerian (*Valeriana officinalis*) is a traditional mood-balancing and calming herb, but unlike chamomile, its effects take about two weeks to become truly visible. Once you feel the calm, it can be quite lasting. Valerian root extract is sedative and calming, but when we are feeling low and tired, it can act as a natural stimulant without the blood pressure-raising effects of caffeine.

Valerian is very useful if you suffer from ongoing anxiety or stress, perhaps at work or in the family. It can also be used to treat insomnia. The common dosage is 300 to 500 mg, but of course you should always seek the advice of a physician when in doubt.

THE MAGIC OF ADAPTOGENS

If the stress is ongoing despite all your efforts to clean up your diet, it's time to take the helping hand that Mother Nature is always ready to offer. Instead of turning to pills, you can try supplementing your diet with adaptogens, natural substances that help the body adapt to stress. They are very effective general body tonics that strengthen the immune, nervous, and glandular systems and bring the body into the much-needed balance. The especial benefit of adaptogens is, like garlic, their ability to re-balance blood sugar. During a stressful event, stress hormones adrenaline and cortisol cause a rapid increase in blood glucose. Once it peaks, the blood glucose rapidly falls to lower than normal levels. Adaptogens help keep blood sugar levels stable.

Siberian ginseng (*Eleutherococcus senticosis*) is a resilient arctic herb with a potent antifatigue, antistress, antiallergenic, and immune-enhancing effect. It works exceptionally well if you are constantly tired and under a lot of pressure at home or at work. Beauty-wise, Siberian ginseng acts as a potent antioxidant and stimulates collagen production.[12] For best results, Siberian ginseng should be taken in two courses, thirty days each, with a two-week interval between them.

Rhodiola (*Rhodiola rosea*) is yet another hardy herb from the Northern hemisphere with a potent immunity-boosting activity. It boosts vitality and energy, enhances resistance to stress and fatigue, and improves the condition of your skin and hair. During a 2012 study, rhodiola was given to people suffering from chronic stress. Scientists noted that the visible therapeutic effect occurred after only three days of treatment.[13] Rhodiola extract is safe and generally well tolerated.

One of the most delicious ways to add rhodiola to your diet is to use it in a Himalayan Health Smoothie. In a blender, combine three or four apricots (pits removed) with two cups of green tea, one teaspoon sea buckthorn extract (in Appendix B you will find some useful online resources to shop for natural ingredients), and a half teaspoon rhodiola tincture. Process until smooth and drink in the morning for a daylong positive mood boost.

Ashwaganda (*Withania somnifera*) is classified in Ayurveda, the ancient Hindu system of medicine, as a rasayana, a group of plant-derived medicines reputed to promote physical and mental health, improve immune function, increase longevity, and revitalize the body. Dubbed "Indian Ginseng," ashwaganda helps enhance energy, achieve a positive state of mind, improves memory and mental performance,[14] and promotes restful sleep—another powerful antiaging tool.

HERBAL NERVE SOOTHERS

There are many herbs and flowers with a proven reputation for effective stress busting. Limeflowers (*Tilia cordata*), skullcap (*Scutellaria lateriflora*), hops (*Humulus lupulus*), passionflower (*Passiflora incarnata*), lemon balm (*Melissa officinalis*), valeriana (*Valeriana officinalis*), and oats (*Avena sativa*) can be taken as teas, tinctures, and tablets. Not only do they help you calm down, but they also help promote a luminous complexion and even improve hair growth.

GET FIT TO RELIEVE STRESS

If you feel tense just thinking about that pair of spandex hot pants you planned to wear at the gym, relax. Exercise is one of the best ways to ease stress and anxiety while giving you a sense of confidence and control over your body and emotions. Physical activity saturates the body with oxygen, so you feel more energized, head to toe. Plus, you are likely to lose a little weight (or not too little, if you stay on track), your skin will regain a lovely glow, and you may begin to enjoy compliments that you look younger and more upbeat.

Some exercise routines are better suited for stress relief than others. One of the best types is interval training, which involves low- to high-intensity exercise interspersed with periods of rest. When you work at a higher intensity even for a short period of time, your body produces ample amounts of feel-good endorphin hormones, which boost your energy, metabolism, and mood. Interval training is extremely easy to do: First, you choose the activity you like—for example, running or cycling. After a short warm up, you increase intensity nearly to the maximum for thirty to sixty seconds, and then reduce intensity allowing your body to relax for two to three minutes. Then repeat the intense stage, following by the relaxing bit. If you jog, try sprinting at your highest possible speed for thirty to sixty seconds, then switch to walking for two to three minutes. Try this routine for twenty to thirty minutes and you will be at astonished how refreshed you will look and feel. Since you do not need to maintain a high intensity for more than a minute at a time, it is easy to stick with this method, and a great way to start a routine.

Other great stress-relieving types of exercise include martial arts, kickboxing (great to let the steam off without actually harming anyone!), circuit training, and of course yoga and pilates. Any sport that gets you closer to the nature such as Alpine walking, mountain biking, skiing, or simply walking in the countryside will bring you into a peaceful, Zen-like state of mind.

Walking is a great way to enjoy a stress-busting power of a workout without the need of expensive gym membership or special equipment. All you need is a pair of walking shoes that are truly multifunctional and some good weather (call me crazy, but I enjoy a brisk walk on a rainy, cold autumn day, with yellow leaves covering the sidewalk, streetlights glowing through the rain, and windows gleaming—you learn to love this kind of stuff when you walk with your child a lot in England).

To me, walking is the ultimate stress-relieving exercise. First, you can truly let you mind wander. You adore the sky, the sunset, the stars; you mind the ground, you smell the flowers, or the freshly cut grass. Breathe in the fresh air using a deep-breathing technique. You look into other people's windows, guessing what kind of joys or troubles are behind those walls and gates. Get away from your problems with a daily walk.

MEDITATE YOURSELF BEAUTIFUL

There is a powerful mechanism that can stop the destruction caused by stress right in its tracks and bring back the calm and peace your body and mind are craving. This mechanism is called meditation. The seemingly simple process of slowing down and breathing deeply activates our body's own natural healing abilities, invigorates the sluggish hypothalamus, and restores pituitary, pineal, and other endocrine glands stymied by chronic stress. In both clinical and nonclinical populations, mindfulness-based meditation has demonstrated benefits for chronic pain,[15] anxiety,[16] depression,[17] fibromyalgia,[18] binge-eating,[19] and psoriasis,[20] as well as improved psychological well-being, immune function, and glycemic control in people with diabetes.[21] This wonderful holistic medicine costs absolutely nothing and is free of any negative side effects.

Roots of meditation can be traced back to prehistoric times. Primitive hunter-gatherers were probably the first practitioners of meditation, as they entered a trancelike state while staring at the fire. Over thousands of years, meditation evolved into a structured practice. Indian scriptures mentioned meditation techniques five thousand years ago, while Buddha became the major meditation guru in 500 BC.

Western Christian meditation stems from the early practice of Bible reading among Benedictine monks called Lectio Divina ("divine reading") and requires no specific postures, although incense and rhythmic repetitions contribute to the deep calming effect on body and mind.

Meditation started to gain popularity in the Western civilization in the 1960s and 1970s as part of "flower power" culture. Very soon, two distinct schools of meditation gained popularity in the West: mindfulness meditation and concentration meditation.

Mindfulness meditation is based on a Buddhist tradition called *vipassana*, one of the world's most ancient meditation techniques. Originally introduced by Gautama Buddha, mindfulness meditation takes your attention inside yourself. You focus your attention on all things passing through the mind but do not allow yourself to judge these things or experience any positive or negative emotions—you simply register the presence of your thoughts and let them go. This meditation technique helps calm anxiety and gradually reroute negative thinking patterns. Transcendental meditation, which is gaining popularity today, requires only twenty minutes of daily practice to achieve a deeply calm, stress-free state of mind.

Focused meditation is part of nearly all religious and spiritual practices. During focused meditation, you focus your attention on a sound, an object, a word, or a body sensation. For example, breathing. Whenever your mind wanders away from its focus, you bring it back to attention on the chosen object.

In the 1970s, the first medical studies confirmed the profound effect of meditation on stress reduction, relaxation, and self-improvement.[22] Since then, the practice has been linked with many long-term psychological and physiological benefits.

Meditation and stress: Meditation literally melts the stress away. Scientists have found that meditation results in lower oxidative stress levels,[23] lower levels of the stress hormone cortisol,[24] and higher melatonin levels.[25] Diaphragmatic breathing is the most helpful element of meditation that lowers stress hormones. It is relaxing and therapeutic, reduces stress, and is a fundamental part of yoga, transcendental meditation, and other meditation practices.[26]

Meditation and sleep: Many people who regularly meditate feel improved energy and tranquility of mind. Researchers have found that people who meditate have higher levels of melatonin compared with people who do not meditate. Scientists found that levels of melatonin in men and women who performed Chinese Original Quiet Sitting, an ancient form of meditation that involves comfortable sitting with hands on one's knees, were "significantly higher" than average.[27] The boost of melatonin, a hormone that helps regulate sleep and also has anti-inflammatory and anticancer activity (you can read more about this important hormone in the next chapter), helps the body to lower the levels of the stress hormone cortisol, as well as dissolve the chemicals that are closely associated with everyday stress. Melatonin is currently used as a sleep remedy, but meditation boosts levels naturally and safely.

Meditation and healthy weight: Stress-relieving exercise and meditation may be more efficient in reducing cholesterol and glucose levels than diet, or exercise alone. During a 2012 study in India, a group of teenage girls with polycystic ovarian syndrome practiced yoga and meditation for one hour per day each day for twelve weeks. Compared to the group who practiced regular physical exercise, the yoga group had lower levels of "bad" cholesterol, and improved glucose, lipid, and insulin values.[28]

Here are some of the other amazing physical benefits of meditation:

- Meditation reduces free radicals in the body, which helps decrease cholesterol levels and promotes younger-looking, glowing skin.[29]
- Meditation slows down biological aging as it increases the levels of sex hormones in older people.[30]
- Meditation improves memory and hearing, often helping eliminate tinnitus (constant ringing in the ears)[31]
- Transcendental meditation and mindfulness-based stress reduction help normalize high blood pressure, studies in 2012 found.[32]

When it comes to skin health, meditation can act as a cheap, completely painless, and effective face-lifting procedure. When we breathe deeply, our skin receives more oxygen and nourishment. When we relax, the tension in facial muscles disappears so face contours appear smoother and firmer. At the same time, rich blood supply helps facial muscles tighten while better blood circulation brings a lovely natural glow to the skin.

Here are some simple meditation techniques, similar to those used in the scientific studies on health effects of meditations:

Clear Mind Meditation
1. Find a quiet and comfortable place indoors or outdoors.
2. Sit in a chair or on the floor keeping your head, neck, and back straight. Relax your hands and feet.
3. Focus on the present moment and put aside all worries, thoughts, or memories.
4. Pay attention to your breathing and notice how the air enters and leaves your body. Feel your belly rise and fall.
5. When worries occupy your mind, simply note that you feel worried but do not allow yourself to spend a second on these emotions. Just make a mental note about them and let them pass away with another breath. Do not judge and do not allow yourself to feel positive or negative. Remain neutral and just breathe.
6. As the time comes to a close, sit for a minute or two, becoming aware of where you are. Get up and continue your day or drift off to sleep, if you meditate in the evening.

For best results, meditate for five minutes twice a day and increase the time spent in peace and quiet for up to one hour.

Walking Meditation

Walking meditation is a Buddhist practice traditionally involving walking down a flat surface that is about twenty-five paces in length (but you can practice this meditation on any surface of any size). The pace of each step is slightly slower than a normal walking pace. You should focus on the actual motion of walking, rather than on your feet. Concentrate your mind on the rise and fall of each foot. Vietnamese walking meditation practice suggests taking one step with each breath. This can be a very slow pace but a powerful way to focus inwards.

1. Before walking, stand for a moment and register how the body is feeling at this very moment.
2. Proceed by calmly and normally pacing out your path with eyes focused on the path five or six feet ahead.
3. Mentally note the complex process of walking—the lifting of the foot, the movement of the foot, the creasing of the sole, and the sound of your feet touching the surface.
4. When reaching the end of the path, focus on the action of turning around and then repeat this process.

You can adapt the walking meditation to any activity you perform daily—from walking up and down the stairs, walking to the bus or train station, or walking your dog. Don't let your mind wander and focus on your body movements to free your mental space from worries and regrets.

Most important, don't forget to eventually go back home!

Are you prone to playing the same worries in your head over and over again? Soothe your mind by writing down the worry the minute it strikes. You can write in a notebook or create a note on your phone. Next, write down the worst possible thing that could happen. It won't erase the worry from your head completely, but it might slow down the worry ride.

Progressive Muscle Relaxation Technique

While not exactly a meditation technique, progressive muscle relaxation (PMR) has a lot in common with focused meditation because it helps reconnect body and mind. PMR focuses on body movements while keeping your mind clear from distractions. By alternately tensing and relaxing the muscles, this technique works to reducing anxiety.

1. To try this relaxation technique, lie down comfortably and loosen any tight clothing.
2. Starting at your ankles, tighten up the muscles for approximately ten seconds and then release for twenty seconds before continuing with the next muscle group.
3. Follow in this sequence: Toes—feet—ankles—thighs—pelvic muscles—abdominal muscles—chest—palms and fingers (clench them in a fist)—arms—shoulders—neck—facial muscles.
4. Keep your eyes closed and concentrate on the sensation of tension and relaxation. Enjoy the feeling of warmth and heaviness after tensing the muscles. For best results, PMR should be practiced at least once a day, ideally during bedtime, for twenty to thirty minutes.

Loving Kindness Meditation

This practice of generating a forgiving, kind attitude toward self and others is a specific meditation practice that can be used both to develop concentration and to fall back in love with your own body and mind. This meditation involves sitting in a quiet place and repeating the phrases below over and over for fifteen to twenty minutes once or twice daily.

1. Sit in a comfortable position, reasonably upright, and relaxed. Fully or partially close your eyes.
2. Take a few deep breaths to settle into your body and into the present moment.

3. Put your hand on your heart for a moment as a reminder to be kind and forgiving to yourself.

4. Form an image of yourself sitting down. Note your posture as if you were seeing yourself from the outside.

5. Now bring your attention inside your body. Feel the pulsation, the slight body movements as you breathe, and how calm and warm your body is. Pay attention to any tense areas, perhaps in your neck, jaw, belly, or forehead.

6. Also notice if you are holding any negative emotions, such as worries, regrets, anxiety, or fears of the future. Understand that every human body bears stress and worry throughout the day.

7. Locate your breathing where you can feel it most easily. Feel how your breath moves in your body.

8. Now offer yourself goodwill because of what you're holding in your body right now. Say the following phrases to yourself, softly and gently:

> *May I be safe.*
> *May I be peaceful.*
> *May I be kind to myself.*
> *May I accept myself as I am.*

9. When you notice that your mind has wandered, return to the words or the experience of discomfort in your body or mind. Gently feel the movement of your breath once again. Go slow.

10. If you are ever overwhelmed with emotion, find a place for it in the physical body and soften that area. When you are comfortable, return to the phrases.

11. Finally, take a few breaths and just sit quietly in your own body. Know that you can return to the phrases anytime you wish.

Gently open your eyes.

When you have gotten the hang of this meditation, you may extend the loving kindness to others in your life, especially those toward whom you feel tension or anger. Imagine the person you are frustrated with and repeat the same phrases: *May he/she be safe, May he/she be peaceful*, and so on. This exercise in compassion will help to ease the tensions in your relationships, and fill you with greater understanding.

HOW TO FIT MEDITATION INTO DAILY LIFE

Meditation can sound daunting at first. Don't let it intimidate you. After all, it is meant to calm you! Start with just five minutes before you drift off to sleep at night, or a simple walking meditation during your usual activities. Then, build up to a more purposeful meditation time every day, starting with just five minutes, and working up to twenty minutes, or half an hour.

Most often, as you finish your meditation, you get caught up in the same mental junk occupying your mind, with all the worries, anxieties, regrets, and expectations. That's why I invite you to treat your meditation sessions not as a "mental spa detox," but rather a part of your personal transformation process.

Take a cue from Buddhist monks and choose a sound that you hear at a regular interval, for example, a church bell, or a sound of an elevator. Take two deep breaths each time you hear this sound. You can also take two deep breaths before you answer a phone call, or open your e-mail.

Do not limit your meditations to your living room floor or your garden, if you are blessed with some peaceful outdoor space. You will be surprised to see many opportunities to meditate as your day goes on. Any repetitive task or a waiting time can be turned into a meditation. You can count your breaths while doing dishes, vacuuming, or sorting your laundry, for example. You can turn exercise into meditation by focusing on your movements, steps, or breathing. Any chore that is automatic in nature will work—but don't try meditation as you drive your car.

THE YOGA WAY TO BEAUTY

Wouldn't you be excited to try a simple exercise routine that helps you lose weight, feel more in control, combat stress, and lift and tone your skin? Achieve it all with yoga. New research suggests that people who practice yoga regularly have lower levels of inflammation-causing compounds in their blood. These compounds, called cytokines, and particularly an inflammation-triggering, obesity-promoting hormone leptin, can lead to heart disease, stroke, arthritis, and diabetes. Studies show that yoga practitioners are less likely than non-practitioners to use medication for metabolic syndrome, mood disorders, inflammation, and pain.[33]

Yoga is extremely helpful to reduce both anxiety and depression. Just two sessions of yoga every week can help you stay in control of your emotions and become more resilient not just to stresses of everyday life, but also to premature skin aging. Add just twenty to thirty minutes of light exercise a day to your yoga practice, and it will make a huge difference to break those anxious or moody cycles. Doing yoga outside is triply rewarding: you get a powerful oxygen boost that reaches every bit of your body; you feel grounded and more in control as you absorb calming nature's imagery; and fresh air invigorates your metabolism, so you move one step closer to the lean, healthy-looking figure of your dreams.

The skin-rejuvenating effect is most profound in yoga inversion poses. Paul Smith recommends two inversions that are so gentle, almost anyone can do them.

Legs Up the Wall Pose: To do Legs Up the Wall Pose (known among yogis as Viparita Karani), lie on the floor with the hips up against the wall and your legs stretched up the wall toward the ceiling.

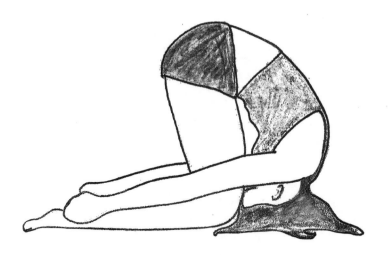

Keep the lower sacrum and tailbone against the floor. For a slightly greater inversion effect, you can put a pillow or folded blanket under the hips. Hold the position for five minutes. If the feet fall asleep, slide the feet down the wall toward the hips, with knees bent over abdomen.

Rabbit (Hare) Pose: For Rabbit Pose (Sasangasana), begin in a child's yoga position kneeling down and then lowering your buttocks to sit on your lower leg and feet. With your arms on the sides, lower your torso on your thighs, as you bring your head down on the floor.

Press your forehead slightly on your knees and extend your arms backward and hold onto the base of your feet. Give your heels a firm hold and then take a deep breath. Roll onto the top of the head, lifting the elbows. The top of the head is on the floor, but more of the body weight is supported by the hands. Hold for twelve slow breaths. At the end of this book, I will suggest several excellent books on yoga that explain this and many other poses in great detail.

If you have a spare minute while sitting at your desk, or watching a movie, you can also try these facial muscle rejuvenating yoga exercises, developed by Paul Smith for this book:

Eye Yoga Exercise: For the eye exercise, hold your head steady, and then shift your eyes seven times each in each direction: right-left; up-down; upper right-lower left; upper left-lower right; clockwise circles; counter-clockwise circles; then touch the thumb to the tip of the nose, focus on the thumb while slowly reaching the arm forward to full arm's length, then focus on the far wall, then back to thumb, then bring thumb to nose—seven times total.

Facial Lift Yoga Exercise: Squeeze the muscles of your face in toward your nose and close your eyes tightly, then open your mouth and eyes widely, spreading out all the muscles of the face. Repeat several times. You can do the facial yoga exercises even when stuck in traffic or waiting in a queue (although the Facial Lift Yoga Exercise may cause a few surprised glances from people nearby). But for the best antistress bang for your fitness buck, head to the park or any other green open space. Even a five-minute workout in the open air is proven to improve your mental fitness. Any open space will give your mood a lift, but green lawns near water are most favorable.

Antistress Massage: Self-massage is the quickest and easiest way to boost your energy levels and dissolve tension at the end of a difficult day. The following massage technique from a massage therapist Suzy Amato will boost your circulation and revive your tense facial muscles. You can add a few drops of the Face Relief Oil below to your fingertips for increased smoothness, and to invigorate the skin.

FACE RELIEF OIL

Essential oils in this recipe are rich in a substance called eugenol, which works as an antistress phytochemical. Eugenol may cause a release of stress–busting neurotransmitters and help combat negative effects of chronic stress.[34] Please keep in mind that eugenol can cause skin sensitivity, so it is very important to cleanse your face thoroughly after massaging if you suspect you may be allergic to any of the recipe components. If you think you may be sensitive to eugenol, please do a patch test first. Dilute the essential oil with base oil (1 drop essential oil to 10 drops of the base oil), and then dab the mixture slightly into the crease of your arm. If no irritation occurs within 24 hours, feel free to explore this recipe.

Ingredients
3.3 oz. (100 ml) cup jojoba or grapeseed oil
5 drops melissa essential oil
2 drops clove essential oil
2 drops nutmeg essential oil
2 drops cinnamon essential oil

Method
Combine all ingredients in a glass (not plastic!) bottle and shake well. Store in a cool dark place for up to 12 months.

1. **Eye Awake.** Sit with your shoulders relaxed, hands placed on your thighs. Close your eyes and firmly press your eyelids together. Do not squint. Count to three, then open your eyes and count to three again. Repeat five times.
2. **Face Tap.** Using fingertips saturated with Face Relief Oil, gently tap your face starting at the forehead and moving down to the cheeks and jaw. You

can also tap your scalp area, which helps release tension and may help promote hair growth.

3. **Cheek Lift.** Using your middle fingers, press firmly into your jaw muscles located under your cheekbones near earlobes. Hold the pressure counting to five, and then relax. Repeat five times.

As you incorporate these simple stress-relieving techniques in your daily beauty routine, remember that the ultimate form of health and beauty is the daily encouragement of positive emotions. Love, compassion, and joy are vital for wellness. On a physical level, they cause your muscles to relax, normalize your breathing, and promote stronger blood flow. The expression of compassion, love, and joy triggers your body to increase the production of serotonin, a natural antidepressant. But the true stress relief is impossible without a good night's sleep. In the next chapter you will learn why your daily slumber is your most powerful antiaging, skin-rejuvenating tool.

Chapter Two Quick Tips

1. If your mood dwindles after you have missed the only parking spot available, or broken a nail before an important date, tackle the issue head on. Remove irritants, relocate your car to another parking garage, and file your nails to perfection. When you **take care of the problem right away**, you enjoy lifted mood, and an added bonus of an accomplishment.

2. Artificial lighting and dark office spaces with no windows can contribute to low moods. If natural sunshine is a luxury for you, for example, in the middle of the winter, **just twenty minutes of being outside in**

natural sunlight can help make a depression-free mind-set a reality.

3. For most of us, taking a break from work or any other activity involves grabbing a coffee and logging in to social networking. If you are feeling overwhelmed, a quick chat with a good friend can be a much better remedy. But if you often socialize with people who complain and whine all the time, it can also contribute to your stress. Instead of worrying about someone else's problems, or reading news (another stress trigger), **get up and take a brisk walk, or close your eyes and listen to classical, lounge, or meditative music.** Most important, never skip your breaks. After just ten minutes of a recharging activity, you will be far more productive than if you plow through the day with no relief.

4. **Make conscious efforts to eliminate sugar, caffeine, or alcohol addictions.** If you are successful at stabilizing your blood sugar levels, you will eventually get off that mood roller coaster that most of us ride on all day.

5. Mind-soothing nutrition will lead to stable physical, mental, and emotional states. **Enrich your diet** with vitamins from the B group, vitamin C, zinc, copper, magnesium, and potassium. Best sources of these nutrients are fresh, wholesome foods, but, if necessary, feel free to add supplements to your daily intake of these stress-relieving nutrients.

6. Consider supplementing with mind-strengthening herbs such as rhodiola or Siberian ginseng, which **help normalize your stress response and reduce the levels of stress-generated free radicals in your body.**

7. **Meditate daily to feel grounded, secure, and less prone to anxiety.** Even ten or twenty minutes a day

can do wonders for your complexion. Choose a meditation technique that fits your personal beliefs and state of mind.

8. Practice facial relaxation massage with soothing oils to **promote the relaxation of facial muscles** and revive a healthy glow.

9. **Yoga is great for your metabolism and overall well-being.** Learn the basics in a studio and try moving your sessions outdoors to absorb more oxygen and soothe your nerves.

THREE

Become a Sleeping Beauty

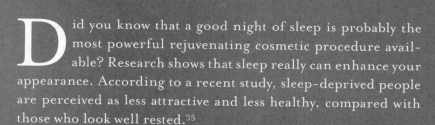

Did you know that a good night of sleep is probably the most powerful rejuvenating cosmetic procedure available? Research shows that sleep really can enhance your appearance. According to a recent study, sleep-deprived people are perceived as less attractive and less healthy, compared with those who look well rested.[35]

Your physical beauty begins in your mind. We all know that worries and anxiety are bad for our health and that you can literally worry yourself sick. But your lack of sleep can bring a whole new host of beauty worries for you. When you don't sleep enough, your body needs to push itself twice as hard to survive on a brink of fatigue. Your body sends energy from already depleted resources where it's needed most: to the heart, brain, muscles, intestines, and endocrine glands. Skin and hair are the last in the list of priorities when our body has access to very limited amount of a recharge time. A lack of healthy circulation to the skin leads to sallow skin, brittle nails, and dark under-eye circles.

When we feel sleepy, our body attempts to put us in a state called "sleep homeostasis." The amount of sleep each of us needs varies from person to person, but adults generally need around seven to nine hours of sleep each night. Any less than that, and you begin accumulating your "sleep debt." This snowballing sleep deprivation has disastrous effect on our looks, including the following:

Red, puffy eyes and increased number of wrinkles around the eyes. As we sleep less, our eyes are more prone to dehydration, which in turn causes micro-injuries to tiny blood vessels in the eye. Result? Redness, puffiness, and dark eye circles as the blood vessels in the lower lid area work hard and often get exhausted "serving" the skin around the tired eye with a fresh supply of oxygen and nutrients.

More blemishes and increased skin dryness. The immune system is weakened without sleep. The number of white blood cells within the body decreases, as does the activity of the remaining white blood cells. The body also decreases the amount of growth hormone produced.

Wider waistline. When sleep deprivation mounts, the ability of the body to metabolize sugar declines, turning more sugar into yet more fat accumulating in the abdominal area. Sleep deprivation reduces levels of leptin, an appetite-depressing hormone. These two changes could lead to abdominal weight gain and contribute to your risk of diabetes.

Sagging facial muscles causing drooping eyelids and deepened nasolabial (nose to corner of the mouth) folds. With chronic sleep deprivation, blood circulation in the facial area is weakened. As a result, facial muscles get fewer nutrients to remain strong and flexible. The continuous frown of tired face becomes permanent, causing even more wrinkles and sagging.

There are less visible but even more dangerous effects of sleep deprivation:

- Increased risk of breast cancer;[36]
- Increase in stress hormones circulating in the blood;[37]

- Increased inflammation, one of the key elements in the development of heart disease;[38]
- High blood pressure, even in young people;[39]
- Reduced short-term memory and concentration;[40]
- Compromised verbal abilities;[41]
- Increased irritability, aggression, and hostility.[42]

Stroke, heart attack, diabetes—these are just some of the diseases that are triggered by sleeping fewer than six hours a night. During a massive European study involving more than twenty-three thousand people over the last eleven years, German scientists found that sleep deprivation was a risk factor in the development of chronic diseases, such as diabetes, heart attack, stroke, and cancer.[43] A similar study conducted by American scientists in 2012 found that people who reported sleeping fewer than six hours a day were more likely to have diabetes than individuals who reported sleeping six to eight hours.[44]

Surprisingly, nearly all of us ignore the simplest tool to determine the best time to doze off: the sun. Our body clock, known as the circadian rhythm, is a twenty-four-hour cycle in biochemical and physiological processes. Disruption of this clock has been implicated in various diseases, ranging from cancer to metabolic syndrome, heart attack, and diabetes.

Circadian rhythms are adjusted by external cues called *zeitgebers*, a term borrowed from German language meaning "time-givers." The main "time-giver" for human beings is daylight. When the sun is up or when we create an artificial sunlight with lamps or candles, our eyes send the information on the lengths of the day and night to the pineal gland, a tiny structure shaped like a pine cone located on the hypothalamus. In response, the pineal secretes the hormone melatonin. Secretion of melatonin peaks at night and nearly stops during the day.

Various studies suggest that shift work that is completely out of tune with the human body clock increases risk of developing cardiovascular and gastrointestinal disorders, some types of cancer including cancers of colon, breast, and prostate, and mental disorders including depression and anxiety. In fact, the International Agency on Research on Cancer (IARC) has recently classified "shift work that involves circadian disruption" as "probably carcinogenic to humans," and calls artificial light during the daily dark period (biological night) as a human carcinogen.[45]

Electric light in the evening messes up our circadian rhythm. Thankfully, the usual lighting in most homes is not enough to severely mess up our inner body clock. But if your lights in the house have a blue tint—such as, for example, fluorescent lights in the kitchen—the damage to your circadian rhythm may be higher. Also, light coming from above has greater impact on our body clock than light coming from the ground up. This is because our brain associates the light from above with a bright sunny day and light from below with a sunset. After dark, dim lamplights kept on low surfaces are best.

When we hear from our grandparents about how they had to get up at four o'clock in the morning to feed the cattle, we reel in horror. But we forget that people who live in tune with nature have the most perfectly set body clock. They fall asleep shortly after the sun goes down. They may get up shortly before the sun goes up, but only during the winter. Such luxury is nonexistent in the civilized world. We go to bed and wake up in disagreement with the natural human circadian rhythm. No wonder we have so much trouble sleeping.

HOW MUCH SLEEP DO WE REALLY NEED?

Sleep deprivation today is almost fashionable. We all know we must get our proverbial eight glasses of water a day, but when it comes to required eight hours of sleep, we give ourselves an enormous amount of slack.

Seven to nine hours of uninterrupted sleep is a classical recommendation when it comes to a healthy sleep. Eight hours of sleep has long been considered the gold standard for pillow time.

But how many of us can honestly say we sleep more than six hours every night? With our relentless online socializing and the availability of late night TV, sleep seems just so boring. Not to mention those lucky individuals who have more exciting things to do at night besides tweeting, chatting, and browsing. And we are not even talking about sleep-deprived new mothers for whom puffy eyes and pallid complexion are not a misery but a badge of honor.

Keep this number in your head: six hours is the minimum you should allow yourself to sleep every day. Anything less than that is just as devastating for your health as smoking, binge drinking, and surviving solely on fast food.

MELATONIN TO THE RESCUE

The quality of our sleep and the rhythmical function of our body clock are governed by the hormone melatonin. Known as the "hormone of darkness," melatonin is a powerful antioxidant, reportedly six to ten times more effective than vitamin E. Lack of melatonin is linked to Alzheimer's[46] and Parkinson's diseases;[47] glaucoma;[48] depressive disorder;[49] breast,[50] prostate,[51] liver,[52] ovarian,[53] and colorectal cancers;[54] and melanoma.[55] As a natural antioxidant with immunity-enhancing properties, this cancer scavenger protects skin cells and mitochondrial DNA and

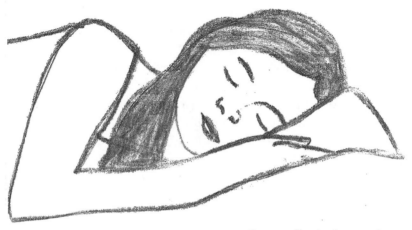

stimulates the release of anti-inflammatory substances such as interleukins and interferon, according to the findings by scientists from the Mount Sinai School of Medicine, New York.[56]

Lack of sleep, nighttime work, frequent wakefulness, and sleeping with a light source in the bedroom all disrupt normal circadian rhythms and may increase the risk of developing cancer. Even a dim light in the bedroom can seep through eyelids and disrupt melatonin release.[57] It has been suspected that women who sleep with a light source in their bedrooms have an increased risk for breast cancer.[58] As a hormone, melatonin counteracts the effects of estrogens. Low levels of melatonin during the night automatically mean higher levels of reproductive hormones fluctuating in the woman's body during the day. As a result, sleep-deprived women or those who must work during the night have higher risk of breast and other hormone-dependent cancers.

Melatonin appears to protect our youthful looks as well. Melatonin helps protect our skin from UV skin damage and also helps the skin to produce another powerful protective substance, vitamin D.

There are several natural ways to preserve melatonin levels. Thankfully, these healthy lifestyle changes also help boost your mood and improve sleep.

Increase your daytime and especially morning sunlight exposure. If the sky is overcast for many days in a row, invest in a light therapy device. You can even get an alarm clock with a built-in light therapy device such as Philips Wake-Up Light, which simulates sunrise to wake you up naturally and pleasantly in the dark mornings.

Eliminate all sources of light in your bedroom. Keep your bedroom dark and quiet. Get rid of night lights, alarm clocks with visible digits, and plug off all electric appliances to avoid those red and green LED lights shining from the corners. If you must keep one alarm clock, turn it toward the wall so less light escapes. Place a towel under the door if the outside light is creeping into your bedroom.

Invest in a high quality blinds to prevent the "visual noise" from the street lights entering your bedroom. Roller "blackout blinds" that completely block the light from the outside are very helpful. Your bedroom should be so dark, you should not be able to see your fingers if you stretch your arm. If you have trouble finding your way in complete darkness (for example, if you need to get out of the room in emergency), paint decorative footsteps leading to the door on the floor with a fine glow-in-the-dark marker. You can also lightly trace furniture edges to avoid bumping into them in the darkness.

BLUE LIGHT EQUALS SLEEPLESS NIGHT

If you are feeling blue, it may mean that your life is overloaded with sneaking blue light. Modern technology emits blue rays from numerous sources: screens of computers, laptops, and phones are all major sources of melatonin-disrupting blue light.[59] Blue light-enriched overhead lights have been shown to increase worker alertness, and are often installed in offices.

Here are some other easy steps to reduce the flow of blue light in your life: Install a free program called F.lux (www .flux.com) on your computer. When enabled, F.lux adapts the hues on your computer to the ambient light, and reduces blue light emissions. Use candles more often. Candles as sources of light are extremely beneficial for your health. The light of candle flames contains virtually no blue light, so there's little damage to your circadian rhythms. Late night TV browsing will dramatically worsen your sleep. If you think that spending a quiet evening in front of the telly will soothe your nerves, reconsider. More likely, it will numb your brain and suppress your melatonin levels thanks to excessive emission of blue rays. Read a book, enjoy a hobby, or meditate instead of wasting your time in front of the TV. Avoid blue, green, or red tinted night-lights. Instead, stick to a dim yellow light for nighttime emergencies. My daughter's favorite night-light is an LED-lighted yellow rubber duck that emits just enough yellow light to soothe and comfort her if she wakes up.

DELICIOUS SLEEPING CURES

The traditional sleep remedy, a cup of warm milk at bedtime, has a lot of scientific studies proving its worth. Milk contains tryptophan, an essential amino acid, which is a precursor of sleep-improving neurotransmitter serotonin. Foods that contain tryptophan and increase serotonin levels include turkey, fish, chicken, cheese, nuts, eggs, and beans. Complex carbohydrates, such as a scoop of brown rice, a handful of nuts, or a few tablespoons of legumes, are essential to helping your brain properly process the tryptophan in protein.

Zinc and magnesium are great not just for your skin and hair condition; these minerals are important for healthy sleep. Magnesium supplements can be used for sleep support. Buckwheat, tomato paste, artichokes, spinach, almonds, cashews, and pumpkin seeds are rich in magnesium, while shellfish (especially oysters), beef, dairy, beans, and oats are excellent sources of zinc. Combine them creatively and eat them at dinner for an easier drift into sleepiness.

Eat a lot of cherries in all forms: fresh, dried, frozen, or as a juice. Cherries are believed to be one of the most concentrated sources of melatonin. Melatonin from food enters the bloodstream and binds to sites in the brain where it helps restore the body's natural levels of melatonin, which can help enhance the natural sleep process. Bananas, corn, and oats also contain melatonin, but in considerably smaller amounts.

CAN LIGHT AT NIGHT CAUSE SKIN CANCER?

The lack of sleep can wreak havoc on your health, but can it actually cause skin cancer? Epidemiologists from Institut Gustave

Roussy in Villejuif, France, suspect that some melanomas may be caused by artificial light.[60] Here's why.

Melanoma rates have been increasing faster than that of any other cancer in recent decades. The main risk factors for skin cancer such as exposure to sunlight, skin tags (nevus) count, phototype (your skin tone), and family history of melanoma may not always explain why this skin cancer is so widespread today. Our sleep patterns, or, to be exact, the lack of sleep patterns may hold the key to the melanoma epidemic.

Studies across the world acknowledge the fact that the increasing use of artificial light-at-night contributed to the increasing breast cancer incidence.[61, 62, 63] As described briefly above, artificial light suppresses the secretion of melatonin, a hormone produced in the dark and inhibited by light, which regulates circadian rhythms. As we already know, melatonin has antioxidant and anticarcinogenic effects that protect the human DNA from mutations. But it also regulates the release of skin pigment melanin in skin cells. Melanin is a natural UV screen inside our skin. The more melatonin is released, the more melanin is produced in our skin, and more natural UV protection from rays we obtain.

People who have skin cancer, especially melanoma, have lower levels of melatonin in their bodies. This could explain why melanoma is common in pilots and aircrews, with increased risk for those traveling with higher exposure to UV rays at higher altitudes. At the same time, office workers exposed to fluorescent lighting also have high risks of melanoma.[64] In this case, blue-tinted fluorescent light that promotes alertness also halts melatonin production. In women, melatonin inhibition increases the risk of melanoma by increasing estrogen levels.

Despite all the supporting evidence, the light-at-night hypothesis has never been directly tested for melanoma. Until the science knows more, your best ally in skin health may not be your sunscreen after all, but your dark, quiet bedroom and regular sleeping hours.

HOW SLEEP HELPS YOU LOSE WEIGHT

Sleep more, weigh less? It could be the perfect slogan for the weight-loss campaign. According to several studies, women who sleep five hours or less per night weigh more on average than those who sleep seven hours. The study found that women who slept for five hours per night were 32 percent more likely to experience major weight gain—gaining 33 pounds or more. But women who slept more are only 15 percent more likely to become obese over the course of the famous sixteen-year Nurses' Health Study that included 68,183 middle-aged women.[65] On average, women who slept five hours or less per night weighed 5.4 pounds more at the beginning of the study than those sleeping seven hours and gained an additional 1.6 pounds more over the next ten years.

"That may not sound like much, but it is an average amount— some women gained much more than that, and even a small difference in weight can increase a person's risk of health problems such as diabetes and hypertension," says lead researcher Sanjay Patel, MD, assistant professor of medicine at Case Western Reserve University in Cleveland, Ohio.

The combination of chronic stress and high-fat, high-sugar diet causes more weight gain than an unhealthy diet would do on its own, according to the research. A brain chemical called neuropeptide-Y (NPY) stimulates appetite and contributes to weight gain. The combination of chronic stress and a high-calorie diet increases the amounts of this neuropeptide in abdominal fat which in turn promotes the growth of new fat cells all over the body. Scientists found that a low-calorie low-glycemic diet that would incorporate daily stress-relieving techniques would help people lose weight more efficiently than would a traditional calorie-restricted weight loss plan.[66]

The reason behind the weight gain could be in female hormones. After a few days of sleep restriction, the hormones that control appetite cause people to become hungrier, so we may hypothesize that women who sleep less might eat more. "But in fact they ate less," Dr. Patel says. "That suggests that appetite and diet are not accounting for the weight gain in women who sleep less." The research did not find any differences in physical activity that could explain why women who slept less weighed more either.

At the moment, the verdict is that sleeping less affects a person's basal metabolic rate, or the number of calories you burn when you rest. Another contributor to weight regulation that has recently been discovered is called non-exercise associated thermogenesis, or NEAT, which refers to involuntary activity, such as fidgeting or standing instead of sitting. It may be that if you sleep less, you move around less too, and therefore burn up fewer calories. Whatever the reason is, those who sleep more have an easier time keeping off unwanted pounds.

HERBAL HELP FOR BEAUTY SLEEP

For most of us, a bowl of oatmeal will prove just as effective as a sleeping pill from the pharmacy, and a magnesium supplement will not only help relax those tense inner muscles you were not aware of, but will help you unwind and relax better than a full-body massage.

When you feel you cannot sleep on your own, here are some natural and herbal remedies that may put you in a healthy, glow-giving, restful slumber:

Oats: Full of vitamin B and calming constituents, oats gently reduces physical and emotional pressure, while nourishing the nervous system. Avena sativa's extract works slowly and it can be taken long-term, ideal for situations where the stress is ongoing. The easiest way to reap on oats' stress reducing action is to eat a bowl of porridge topped up with honey every evening at bedtime. This combo will knock you out in no time!

Valerian: Valerian contains a relaxing substance known as valerinic acid. For this reason, it has traditionally been used to reduce sleeplessness, tension, and muscle spasms. Valerian also has a sedating effect on mind and body and is often combined with hops (see below). If you decide to take valerian for your stress, please keep in mind that it can take up to two weeks to show any visible results, but once you see them, you will not know how you coped without valerian, as its action is so mild yet so natural and holistic. I attribute my first breakthrough from acne to valerian, as I believe it helped soothing my stress-induced blemishes. Stress-related eczema can also be diminished with regular intake of valerian extract, along with natural skincare and stress-reducing exercises such as pilates and yoga.

Hops: Well known as an important ingredient for beer, hops, a type of flower from an herbaceous perennial plant, has a long history of another traditional use. It is a climbing plant, containing substances known as hurnulones and lupulones, which have calming effects on the body's nervous system.

Sage: It is not only worry and stress that can disturb sleep. Menopausal night sweats can also cause sleepless nights for women and this restlessness can affect the sleep of their partners too. Sage has been used traditionally for excessive sweating and hot flushes during the menopause.

Naturally boosting melatonin levels helps improve sleep without the need of sleeping pills. Melatonin contains in many plants including feverfew (*Tanacetum parthenium*), and St. John's Wort (*Hypericum perforatum*). These herbs are available as supplements and herbal teas. Try them for at least a month to see any difference they make on your sleeping habits. Calcium, magnesium, vitamin B6, and niacinamide help improve the quality of sleep, which in turn allows the brain to release more melatonin.

Here is a time-tested natural sleep aid that helps soothe the mind and promote a restful sleep.

LAVENDER & MILK FOOT BATH

Lavender is a well-known nerve soother. Added benefit: your tired feet will feel silky and smooth after this bath. You can also place a tissue with a few drops of lavender on your pillow to help you sleep.

Ingredients
5 drops lavender essential oil
½ cup milk

Method
Add the lavender oil to the milk and pour it in the warm water in a basin. Soak your feet five to ten minutes.

Silk bed linen may be costly but it has lots of beauty benefits. Sleeping on silk pillowcases may help diminish so-called "sleep lines," wrinkles on the face and neck which may form or deepen due to pressure between our face and our pillows or sheets. Natural silk is hypoallergenic, antibacterial, and antifungal, and does not harbor dust mites as traditional fabrics do. If you cannot afford buying a full silk bed linen set, at least try silk pillowcases. There are also duvet covers with silk filling.

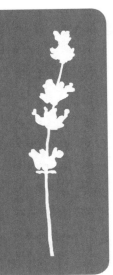

TOP TEN FOODS FOR SLEEP

1. *Oats*
2. *Pumpkin and sesame seeds*
3. *Cherries*
4. *Shellfish, especially scallops and oysters*
5. *Almonds*
6. *Buckwheat*
7. *Artichokes*
8. *Turkey*
9. *Cheese (in moderation)*
10. *Beans*

START SLEEPING BETTER TODAY

Frightened by how behind you are on restful sleep? The only solution is to try to catch up on your sleep on a consistent basis. It sounds boring, but it works.

You will know it when you have slept off the sleep debt you have accumulated over years of chronic sleep deprivation. Your skin will regain its glow and tone, and your eyes will be less puffy and the under-eye area will be less dark and wrinkled.

If you "force" yourself to sleep at least seven hours every night for just seven days, miracles will start to happen. You will suddenly notice that your clothes are less pinching in the waist area. Maybe that stubborn "spare tire" around your midriff will become less stubborn. Your cheeks may be less puffy, your skin less droopy, your hair less limp. And there are lots of "mores" in the good sleep story. For starters, your skin will become firmer. Your hair will have more gloss. You will feel more energy throughout the day without gulping mugs of coffee or caffeinated sugar-laden soft drinks. You will suddenly realize that life is more than television and online socializing.

Some of the "sleep-better" recipes are not suitable for extreme life situations such as having a new baby. My personal recipe for breaking that sleepless rut when I was dealing with a teeny-weeny poor sleeper was to take her outside, rain or snow, night or day, midnight, or early morning. We just stepped outside, wrapped in comfy warm clothes if necessary, and wandered around the garden or along nearby quiet streets. Ten minutes later, both of us would be dozing off on the move. Twenty minutes later, we would be fast asleep in our beds. Do as you wish, as long as it helps you unwind and becomes sleepy. Meditate, soak your jagged nerves in a fragrant bath, read a funny book—just don't jump on the trampoline or hit the treadmill, and keep away from the TV, tablet, or a computer.

I am living proof of the benefits of reducing your sleep debt. Back home in the civilized world, I used to work six hours a day at the office, and five hours in the late evening after putting my daughter to bed, surviving on five hours of sleep (interrupted once or twice) per night. I would drag myself out of bed every morning, and gulp mugs of strong coffee in order to stay alert on a frozen mountain road during a morning school run. Yet, every year when we joined my mother's holiday retreat on the Black Sea, I would catch on my sleep, and it always worked wonders. Right after enjoying three or four nights of a blissfully undisturbed eight hours of sleep, I would brim with new ideas for my skincare and books, and physically I would feel at the top of the world. I would marathon swim; I would hike in the wilderness; I would play competition-level tennis for several hours. Even though my days were shorter by two or three hours, I was living my life a whole lot better than I would if I were skimming it with my eyes half open and my brain half numb.

Sleep is designed to restore us. During the night, tissues are repaired; organs rest or work hard flushing out toxins. Our mind also uses the sleep to filter everything that has happened that day, eradicating the useless, saving the beneficial for us to use later on. "Sleeping on it" is a great technique—for me, it's imperative to postpone an important decision until the "morning after," for many wonderful ideas spring to mind if you give it a chance to take a break from your daily burdens. To give your mind a much-needed rest, you actually need to sleep—staring at the ceiling all night just doesn't have the same effect.

Chapter Three Quick Tips

1. When sleep is disturbed we can find our brains struggling to cope, our memory slipping, increased feelings of anxiety, poor concentration, muscle fatigue, dull skin, and blood-shot eyes. **Aim for seven to hours of sleep every night.**

2. To start reaping the benefits of a beauty sleep, **re-establish your internal clock by sticking to a regular bedtime schedule.** Even if your schedule varies, set a regular bedtime and wake up time. Try to maintain this even on the weekends. The ideal time to go to bed is before midnight. An hour of sleep before midnight will do your health more good than three hours of fogged sleep after midnight.

3. **If you drink coffee, teas, or other caffeinated beverages, try cutting back,** or at least not having any during the afternoon or later.

4. **Avoid alcohol.** Although it may make you drowsy, it also makes you waken more easily later on, maybe to fret about something that may never happen, or just to roam through your regular nighttime fears. If you often wake up at night, try drinking more

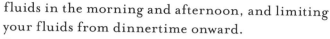

fluids in the morning and afternoon, and limiting your fluids from dinnertime onward.

5. **Regular exercise** can promote good night's sleep. Late afternoon activity seems to be best, but avoid exercising within three hours of bedtime.

6. Mattresses and pillows do not last forever. Check yours to **make sure they are giving you the support you need.**

7. **Calcium and magnesium supplements at bedtime promote healthy sleep** and recharge your body's energy supply.

8. **Cherries are rich in natural "nightcap" hormone melatonin,** which acts as a powerful antioxidant, cancer protector, and skin rejuvenator.

9. **Create a sleep routine that you stick to every night,** to indicate to your brain that it is time to sleep. This provides an excellent change to incorporate some of the lifestyle and beauty tips throughout this book. For instance, an hour before you want to be snoozing, wash your face and give yourself a soothing massage with an essential oil. Then, meditate for fifteen minutes before sitting down to read or do something else you enjoy that is calming, such as knitting. Then get into bed and doze!

10. **Keep your bed, or, ideally, your entire bedroom, for sleep only.** Do not keep your computer in your bedroom. Do not pile your bedside table with assignments from work. Do not watch TV before trying to go to sleep. Make your bed a safe haven, where the stresses of life are not allowed to enter, and peace and quiet prevail.

11. Don't eat late dinners or late-night snacks. Ideally, **finish eating three hours before bedtime.**

FOUR

Eat Yourself Beautiful

Next time you lose your precious beauty sleep over some astronomically priced cleansing device or the latest wrinkle-erasing cream, consider this: some of the most effective beauty tools can be found right on the shelves of your fridge and kitchen cupboards. From crunchy apples to juicy fish fillets, your food has a profound effect on the condition of your skin, nails, and hair. Add to the recipe the contents of your kitchen cupboards, with all their nuts, legumes, honey, oils, and spices, and you have all you need for the smooth, glowing, age-resistant skin and a full mane of hair.

Our looks reflect what's going on inside our bodies, so if there's eye puffiness, skin dryness, brown spots, or acne, then it's time to look within. Correcting your diet is the quickest way to improve your skin and hair. Every part of the body is self-repairing, self-maintaining, and constructed exclusively using "building blocks" from our diet. The sad truth is that skin is the last body organ to benefit from even the cleanest, nutrient-rich diet consisting of fresh, natural foods. Vital nutrients first go to the brain, muscles and internal body organs, while skin humbly waits at the end of the queue for its portion of glow-boosting, age-rewinding nutrients.

The skin-boosting diet is based on nutrient-rich fresh, minimally processed foods and an ample intake of water. In fact, water is the least expensive yet probably most effective beauty tool at your disposal. Water helps carry nutrients to skin cells and to flush toxins. To improve skin's eliminating functions and help rehydrate and plump the skin from the inside, two liters (of good quality noncarbonated water or simply filtered tap water is the average amount you need each day. If your diet is on the fatty side, you need even more than that. Remember that fresh fruit and vegetables are rich sources of water as well as the valuable nutrients concentrated in their cells. Water in fresh fruit and vegetables is released gradually, as the food is digested, while water drunk by the glass simply passes too quickly resulting in frequent trips to the toilet, rather than profound skin hydration.

It is best to drink one full glass of water, possibly with a splash of lemon juice and a teaspoon of organic honey, immediately upon waking, and the rest of your water intake should take place between meals—this helps suppress the appetite and also does not hinder food digestion during meals. Herbal teas and diluted fruit juices are great skin hydrators too. Ginger, chamomile, and nettle infusions have calming and detoxifying properties that help clear and refine your skin. Here's a lovely simple recipe of a skin clearing tea that also helps diminish eye puffiness:

• •

SKIN DETOX TEA

Ingredients
2 sachets (tea bags) of peppermint tea
2 sachets of chamomile tea

2 cardamom pods

1 teaspoon dried orange peel (optional)

Method

Combine all ingredients in a coffee filter and add boiling water. You may sweeten this tea with honey or stevia. Enjoy up to 3–5 cups daily.

● ●

PROTEIN SKIN BOOST

Our skin remains tough and resilient thanks to protein, which helps repair the skin just as any other organ in the body. As we age, skin cell turnover slows down, but with adequate protein intake, our skin and hair receive enough amino acids to function in a youthful mode. Protein also maintains skin's supportive scaffolding, collagen and elastin fibers hidden deep in the dermis and in the joints too. If you eat animal protein, choose organic chicken and turkey to benefit from healthier fats and to diminish antibiotic and pesticide residue found in conventionally farmed birds. Organic, free-range eggs are amazing sources of skin-rejuvenating amino acids and lecithin, essential for healthy hair—but remember that eggs can also raise your cholesterol, so stick to one or two at a time, as opposed to the five-egg omelets found in diners. You can also add a little liver to your diet—it's a rich source of vitamin A, a powerful anti-ager. But avoid liver or vitamin A supplements if you are pregnant or thinking about having a baby. Vegetarian sources of skin-friendly protein include seeds, nuts, beans, quinoa, chick peas, and lentils. Fish is an ideal beauty-boosting protein, as it contains very beneficial essential omega-3 fatty acids. Let's talk about this potent wrinkle and acne fighters in more detail.

One of the most valuable types of protein for our skin is collagen. It's the most abundant protein in the body counting up to 90 percent of the skin's volume. Starting at age twenty-five, the amount of collagen in our bodies gradually diminishes due to sun exposure, a less-than-healthy lifestyle, nutritional deficiencies, and general body toxicity that generates free radicals which damage collagen. Thankfully, we can slow down the destruction of this amazing protein that not only prevents skin wrinkling and sagging, but also keeps our joints flexible and resilient.

The most reliable way to protect collagen from destruction is to consume ample amounts of antioxidants in a natural, bioavailable form. Antioxidants that protect collagen include zinc, vitamin C, vitamin E, and coenzyme Q10. Vitamin C helps the body maintain healthy tissues and improves overall immunity. Thankfully, you don't have to gulp pints of orange juice to maintain glowing skin. Vitamin C can be found in kiwis, red peppers, guavas, strawberries, Brussels sprouts, grapefruits, and mangoes. The recommended daily allowance (RDA) for adult men is 90 mg and for adult women its 75 mg. For example, a medium-sized kiwi fruit contains 74 mg of this essential beauty vitamin, blackcurrants contain up to 200 mg per cup of berries, and acerola cherries contain a whopping 1,677 mg in just one cup!

If you wish to add a vitamin C supplement to your daily beauty routine, look for time-released forms because vitamin C is washed out from the body within four hours. Instead of a once-a-day horse pill of ascorbic acid, choose an oil-soluble form of vitamin C called ester-C or l-ascorbic acid.

Vitamin E is another top beauty vitamin that not only preserves the collagen but also helps maintain healthy skin cell membranes so they can better hold onto water and nutrients. The RDA for vitamin E is 15 mg a day for adults, but in natural form this vitamin is tricky to obtain because vitamin E—rich foods are also very calorific, with high oil content. Vitamin E is abundant in avocados, sunflower seeds, pine nuts, hazelnuts, almonds, turnip greens, peanut butter, wheat germ, and tomatoes, which are also a source of the antiaging, cancer-preventing phytonutrient lycopene. Vitamin E supports the antioxidant action of vitamin C and prevents it from escaping the body too quickly, so it's a good idea to combine both beauty vitamins in one meal—for example, snack on strawberries and nuts or dress the tomato salad with olive or sunflower oil.

Since collagen is made up from eighteen amino acids, of which glycine and proline are most plentiful, eating foods that naturally boost levels of these amino acids may help preserve collagen.[67] Glycine and proline are naturally contained in chicken skin, crab meat, lobster, crayfish, and scallops. A rich vegetarian source of collagen-boosting amino acids is seaweed spirulina, which can be added to juices and smoothies.

To help your skin hold onto its collagen reserves, you may also consider supplementing with marine collagen. Derived from salmon skin and cartilage, animal collagen has shown potential to inhibit collagen loss in animal studies, improve wound healing, and act as an antioxidant.[68] Look for hydrolyzed marine collagen, or marine collagen peptides from reliable supplement manufacturers.

BEAUTIFUL OILS

Essential fatty acids found in vegetable oils, nuts, and seeds are vital to nourish the skin and keep it strong and irritation free. Cold-pressed oils such as olive, sunflower, rice bran, and flaxseed are the best sources of anti-inflammatory "omegas." The easiest way to reap the beauty-boosting benefits of these oils is to dress your salads with a simple mixture of cold-pressed oil, some fresh lemon juice, and maybe garlic and herbs.

Extra virgin olive oil is perhaps the most beneficial oil for your skin and hair, and it is widely available. Olive oil has been shown to reduce levels of low-density cholesterol levels and to reduce blood pressure as well. Studies suggest that regular olive oil consumption may reduce your risk of certain cancers. There is some evidence suggesting that olive oil, as part of a Mediterranean diet rich in fiber and fresh vegetables, could greatly reduce breast cancer risk.[69] When applied topically, olive oil provides very weak sun protection (it cannot substitute for sunscreen, but it may suffice to protect your hair from being discolored by the sun). And of course, you can use olive oils alone to moisturize your hair, skin, and nails as it is rich in antioxidant phytochemicals and skin-softening lipids.

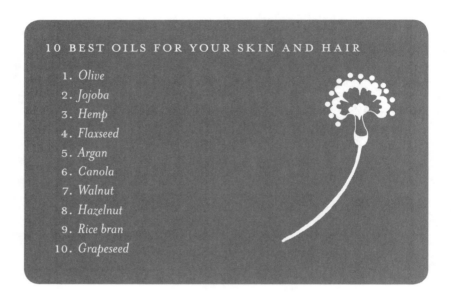

10 BEST OILS FOR YOUR SKIN AND HAIR

1. *Olive*
2. *Jojoba*
3. *Hemp*
4. *Flaxseed*
5. *Argan*
6. *Canola*
7. *Walnut*
8. *Hazelnut*
9. *Rice bran*
10. *Grapeseed*

The following foods will provide you with enough essential omega-3 fatty acids to keep your skin and hair glowing, when taken daily:

- 1 teaspoon flaxseed oil or 1 tablespoon raw ground flaxseeds (not toasted)
- 1 cup soybeans or edamame beans
- ½ cup walnuts or hazelnuts
- 1 tablespoon extra virgin olive or hemp oil

To maintain your skin in top condition over the years, make a gradual shift toward a diet rich in high-quality oils. Experiment with various nut butters, such as walnut or almond, on your toast or crackers. Make spreads and sandwich fillers with avocado, nuts, seeds, and tofu and generously add seeds and nuts to your salads and cereals. Nut butters made from peanuts, almonds, and cashews are rich sources of healthy monounsaturated fats and are also good sources of fiber as well as important vitamins such as B vitamins, folic acid, and glow-boosting vitamin E. You can spread nut butters on toast and even add them to soups and stews to boost protein and antioxidant content. Choose nut butters that are low in added salt and sugar.

To fry or sauté your foods, use organic olive and canola oils and do not heat your oils too much. If you can see the oil smoking, it is not good for you anymore. The following oils survive heat the best: olive, coconut, canola (make sure to buy organic as most canola is genetically modified), peanut, sunflower, and safflower oils.

THE NUTRITIONAL FACELIFT

A healthy, balanced diet is obviously essential for glowing skin, but including some of the well-studied wrinkle-busting foods will help reveal smoother, better-toned, softer skin—without the astronomical price tag or excessive toxin exposure.

Healthy skin and simple carbohydrates such as white sugar and white flour are simply incompatible. Sugar, especially when ample amounts of sunlight are available, damages the supportive tissue of the skin by cross-linking collagen and elastin in an irreversible process called glycation. The more sugar you consume, the more wrinkles you get.[70] "This process is accelerated in all body tissues when sugar is elevated and is further stimulated by ultraviolet light in the skin," writes dermatologist Dr. William Danby of Dartmouth Medical School in Hanover, New Hampshire. Sugar not only destroys your resilient and springy collagen and elastin fibers, it also triggers low-grade inflammation, which leads to skin irritations and blemishes. Therefore, avoiding or at least limiting sugar in your diet may be the best way to maintain the healthy spring and resilience in your skin. For best results, eliminate not only obvious sources of sugar such as sweets, pastries, cakes, ice cream, and chocolate, but also wheat, which ferments into sugar, and alcohol, which contains a lot of sugar. Eliminating sugar from your diet is definitely less toxic than Botox injections and less painful than a facelift, and may bring results that are just as dramatic.

Instead of sugar, sweeten things up with honey. Truth is, it is highly calorific—but it is a fantastic, nutrient-rich alternative to sugar and sugar products. Opt for a local, unprocessed variety or New Zealand Manuka honey. Eating local honey may also help ease hay fever—but make sure you are not allergic to bee products first. A teaspoon of honey stirred into a large glass of water with an added squeeze of a lemon makes an easy detox drink. It boosts up your skin glow, detoxifies the liver, and jump-starts your metabolism so you use up your calories from food more efficiently.

The second big change you can make is to replace simple carbs with complex carbohydrates, which provide more body-cleansing fiber and sustained energy release. Complex carbs include whole grains such as brown rice, oats, millet, barley, lentils, quinoa, buckwheat, and whole wheat, as well as root vegetables, legumes, squash, and pumpkin. Not only do they contain lots of fiber, but they also provide essential minerals such as bone-strengthening magnesium and antioxidant selenium.

Selenium is extremely important to maintain the youthfulness of your skin as well as minimize the risk of skin cancer. Skin-wise, it helps thicken the skin and reduce sun spots and other signs of long-term sun damage. Along with vitamins C and E, selenium wards off free radicals that damage the skin's DNA and may lead to skin cancer. As selenium prevents and in some ways reverses the skin damage by UV rays, it reduces the thickening of the skin caused by excessive sun exposure, so the skin remains smooth, elastic, and soft. Selenium can be found in nuts, seaweed, and sesame seeds, but you can also top levels of this mighty antioxidant with supplements. For best results, your antiaging skin supplement should contain generous amounts of selenium lycopene, lutein, beta-carotene, and a natural source of vitamin E.

Molecules of silica (silicon) give strength and hardness to skin, hair and nails. Silica is the most abundant mineral in Earth's crust. In the human body, silica is part of some of the most resilient human tissue such as arteries, tendons, eyes, joints, and skin. Silica helps form collagen as it is part of the collagen-building amino acid proline; it also forms keratin and hyaluronic acid, vitally important constituents of a healthy skin. As a mineral, silica is a quartz crystal, so it has very definite crystalline structure. Homeopaths believe that silica promotes wound healing and reduces scars, which may be due to silica's ability to penetrate deep into the dermis and "patch things up" with increased collagen formation. It also helps draw toxins out of the skin. Silicate clays montmorillonite and kaolin are great for skin detoxification and rejuvenation. You can also boost levels of silica in your body naturally with silica supplements or by increasing the amount of fiber in your diet. Whole grains, nuts, seeds, vegetables, and mushrooms are great sources of readily available silica to nourish our skin and hair.

Zinc is another essential component of healthy skin, but don't think its only task is to keep you pretty. Zinc participates in the creation of vital enzymes that regulate each and every function and reaction of our bodies. Unfortunately, our ability to absorb this vital metal reduces with age. Zinc is also essential for a healthy hormonal balance, lactose digestion, liver health, DNA maintenance, strong bones, tough immune system, and smooth kidney function—to name just a few of its functions. Zinc also helps the body make good use of vitamin A coming from various sources, and this helps zinc and vitamin A work together to maintain your glowing complexion. Make sure you add zinc to your multivitamin ration as quickly as possible; this metal is one of the mightiest antioxidants helping you stay beautiful.

For ages, humans obtained zinc from grains, dairy, and meat, but technological progress depleted our soils of this vital element.

These days, fish and crustaceans are better sources of zinc than meats and dairy. Oysters, shellfish, and coldwater fish, especially herring, contain exceptional zinc levels. Animal sources, such as eggs and liver, contain fairly high levels of zinc but still lower than those found in seafood.

Zinc is better absorbed from animal foods rather than plant sources, so if you are a vegetarian you should think about supplementing your diet with zinc in the form of zinc citrate or zinc gluconate. Whole wheat, rye, oats, and beans are good sources of zinc. Pecans and Brazilian nuts are also good sources of zinc for vegetarians and omnivores. You can also consume zinc from cooking liquids, especially from vegetables. Zinc is readily soluble in water, so when you cook your grains or beans, much of the zinc is lost in water. Think twice about discarding that water from boiled beans or Brussels sprouts! Save it to make a batch of soup or a sauce for your next meal; cooking your rice or pasta in the water where your vegetables cooked not only saves time, but also adds flavor and nutrients to your meal.

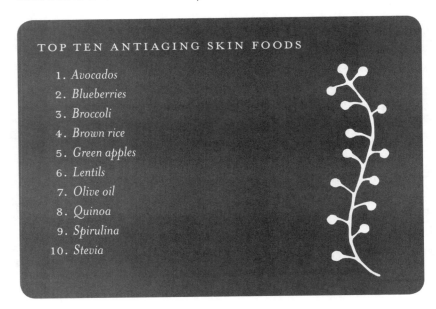

TOP TEN ANTIAGING SKIN FOODS

1. *Avocados*
2. *Blueberries*
3. *Broccoli*
4. *Brown rice*
5. *Green apples*
6. *Lentils*
7. *Olive oil*
8. *Quinoa*
9. *Spirulina*
10. *Stevia*

THE BEAUTY OF FIBER

There is yet another reason to embrace complex carbs: they are incredibly rich source of another beauty essential, namely, fiber. "Roughage" is crucial for healthy complexion and trim, flat tummy as it binds to toxins and helps eliminate them from the body before they hit the bloodstream and reach other vital organs. Less stress for your liver means clear, healthy skin and less abdominal fat as your liver is the main organ of detoxification. Since fiber cannot be broken down by enzymes, it travels through the intestines, grabbing up all the dirty bits along its way. A sluggish, stagnant colon causes your belly to protrude and your skin to work double shifts eliminating toxins. And there's yet another reason to eat lots of fiber-rich foods: this natural scrub for your intestines also helps reduce excessive levels of estrogen hormones in the body, which may help maintain glowing complexion and reduce the risk of breast[71] and uterine[72] cancers.

Choosing the right type of fiber for your body can be tricky. If you are not accustomed to ample amounts of fiber, then "hard" fibers, such as cellulose found in wheat bran and psyllium husks, can clog up your colon and cause even more trouble. To avoid this, you should slowly teach your body to operate under extra fiber weight with soluble fibers, such as pectin, gums, and mucilage, which form gels in the colon and have a gentler yet effective cleansing effect. Pectin is contained in apples, guavas, quince, plums, gooseberries, oranges, and other citrus fruits. Gums are present in oat bran, oatmeal, beans, and sesame seeds, while ample amounts of mucilage can be found in psyllium fiber.

Introducing more fiber is quite easy. An apple a day may not keep the doctor away, but three apples are more likely to do the trick. All nuts, seeds, and whole grain cereals such as barley, buckwheat, quinoa, millet, and whole wheat supply our bodies with ample amount of fiber along with vitamin E, magnesium, and other minerals and vitamins contained in their unprocessed form. For other foods, fiber and sugar content are interlinked.

Because of the food particle size, chocolate has lower glycemic index than brown rice—yet, of course, brown rice provides our bodies with much more fiber than chocolate! With other high-fiber foods, there's a battle between water soluble and insoluble fiber. For example, barley has a lower glycemic index and therefore lower potential to cause skin problems than whole wheat. So which sources of fiber are most beneficial?

When choosing natural sources of fiber, low glycemic index types should be your first option. The World Health Organization recommends that you take up to 40 grams of fiber daily. Barley, rye, peanuts, soy beans, and other legumes have relatively low glycemic index and therefore provide a good balance between fiber and sugar intake.

Fiber comes as a supplement too. If needed, for best results, take your supplements with a probiotic or after eating a natural yogurt enriched with milk bacteria, followed by two glasses of pure water.

However, be careful of fiber supplements. Sometimes too much fiber can cause as much problems as too little. When you overload your body with fiber, you risk depleting your stocks of iron, calcium, and zinc, which can be disastrous not just for your skin but for your overall well-being. To avoid this, the best option is to go easy on supplements, especially wheat bran, and eat instead a lot of various natural foods that are rich in fiber. Unfortunately, as beneficial as plant fiber can be to health, there's nearly always a side effect of excessive gassiness. Gas production, as unpleasant as it seems, is actually quite healthy: it protects the gut from carcinogens, speeds up bowel function and even improves the health of cells that line colon walls. But when we eat too many fiber-rich carbohydrates (most often, legumes), the colon starts being loud. One of the options is to reduce the amount of gas-producing beans and members of the cabbage family in one meal and to never eat them together. I also found that eating small-sized legumes such as lentils is less problematic for the colon than larger varieties such as white, kidney, or lima beans. If you really must use your white beans for a specific recipe, say, baked beans or a casserole, soak them overnight—this simple trick greatly reduces the gas factor. And remember that when you embrace fiber-rich foods, your intestinal flora will prosper, which, in turn, improves your body's ability to deal with gas-producing foods without causing your belly to explode. Sooner or later your body will learn how to cope with beans or cabbage without becoming explosive.

TURN BACK THE CLOCK WITH ANTIOXIDANTS

When planning a weekly shopping list, aim for antioxidants. Environmental pollutants, smoking, drinking, a nutritionally deficient diet, and excessive sun exposure all generate free radicals—oxygen molecules with one electron which allows them to latch onto every molecule available. As long as they can hold onto the molecule, the destruction by oxidation begins. When our bodies become oxidized too quickly, they begin to age prematurely, with all the unpleasant side effects that come along with that. It is estimated that nearly one-third of all cancer deaths in the United States could be prevented through better diet, especially by increasing consumption of fruits and vegetables rich in antioxidants.[73]

Not only are antioxidants vitally important to ward off premature aging, they support your whole body's functioning, which, in turn, brings a healthy glow that no bronzer is able to fake.

Some of the most important dietary antioxidants are green tea polyphenols, curcumin, genistein from soy, resveratrol from grapes, and lycopene from tomatoes and carrots.

When consumed regularly, they add to the mighty punch against cancers of the skin, prostate, breast, lung, and liver. They also keep your skin glowing and hair flowing no matter your age.

Fruits and vegetables with the most intense colors are highest in age-rewinding phytochemicals. It makes your life a bit easier as you approach the fresh produce aisle. Beetroot, aubergines, all kinds of berries, broccoli, spinach, sweet potato, kale, pumpkins, and butternut squash—as long as the produce is brightly colored, grab it and place it into your basket. No guesswork required!

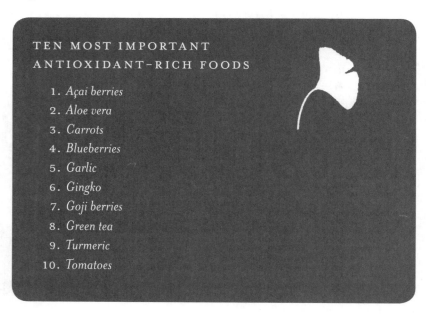

TEN MOST IMPORTANT
ANTIOXIDANT-RICH FOODS

1. *Açai berries*
2. *Aloe vera*
3. *Carrots*
4. *Blueberries*
5. *Garlic*
6. *Gingko*
7. *Goji berries*
8. *Green tea*
9. *Turmeric*
10. *Tomatoes*

There are thousands of antioxidant combinations in brightly colored fruits and vegetables, and some antioxidants exist only in a single type of plant. Some of them are especially helpful in achieving a glowing, resilient complexion.

Green tea contains antioxidant polyphenols that help prevent skin damage from excessive sun exposure. In this way, green tea can help prevent skin cancer if taken orally[74] or applied topically as a toner or when included in a moisturizer.[75] You can strengthen the sun protective potency of your sun cream by lightly misting your skin with green tea and allowing it to soak in and dry before applying the moisturizer. Just one or two cups of green tea daily will strengthen your skin's defenses against the sun.

Milk thistle is a well-studied antioxidant herb that contains a unique flavonoid, called silymarin. It is commonly taken by people with liver diseases, but recent studies show that silymarin also helps prevent skin cancer by neutralizing free radicals generated by sun exposure or less-than-pristine environment.[76]

Aloe vera contains enzymes that protect skin cell membranes from free radical damage. Perhaps this explains the soothing and healing effect that aloe vera gel has on damaged or sunburnt skin. There are many varieties of aloe vera juices in health food stores. Aloe vera juice has a very bitter taste, so it is usually sweetened with honey or agave syrup. For skincare applications, the unsweetened variety is better because it will be less sticky.

Coenzyme Q10 (CoQ10) helps maintain youthful energy production in all cells of the body, especially in the heart, brain, and skin. This vital enzyme can be obtained naturally from oily fish such as mackerel, sardines, and salmon, or from whole grains. You can also take it as a supplement.

Lycopene is a carotene found in tomatoes but also in other red fruits and vegetables, such as red carrots, watermelons, and papayas. Lycopene is simply brilliant when it comes to skin protection against harmful sun exposure. When our skin is exposed to sunlight, it immediately suffers from photodamage and oxidative stress, which may lead to skin cancer. When applied to the skin or taken as a food, lycopene decreases inflammation, protects skin DNA, and reduces skin thickness, which is often a result of sun damage.[77] The antioxidant activity of skin treated with lycopene was found to be ten times higher than untreated skin. Tomato paste is the best source of lycopene, along with carrot and tomato juices. You can also take a lycopene supplement—start taking it daily at least one month before your summer vacation to greatly diminish the risk of sunburn and long-term skin damage.

FEED YOUR HAIR AND NAILS

Our hair and nails are the last to receive nutrients from food and supplements, but thankfully there are several phytonutrients and minerals that can make the "mane" difference to your hair. If our body doesn't receive enough of them, hair growth can slow down and our locks lose that gorgeous luster.

Regular intake of vitamins A, B, C, D, and E is very important for natural development of scalp and hair bulbs, healthy protein metabolism, and tissue growth. But when it comes to hair, two elements are exceptionally important. One of them is zinc. Zinc may improve hair growth, strengthen hair bulbs, and prevent hair from falling out too quickly. Eggs are building blocks of glowing skin and hair, so make sure to eat an egg a day to keep the wig away. Make a small omelet, and throw in handfuls of fresh herbs from the garden or dried from the supermarket. So keep your zinc levels topped up, not just with eggs, but with pumpkin seeds, sunflower seeds, sweet potatoes, pine nuts, and oysters.

Of all B vitamins, biotin (vitamin B7) is especially important for healthy hair growth. Biotin has hair-stimulating effect and may even slow down hair graying or baldness. When babies do not receive enough biotin from their milk, they may develop cradle cap, crusty yellow patches around the scalp and eyebrows. Biotin also helps improve eczema, dry skin, rashes and red, sore eyes. Adults need up to 30 mcg of biotin a day. This vitamin is abundant in egg yolks, brewer's yeast, whole grain rice, nuts, tomatoes, onions, and cabbage.

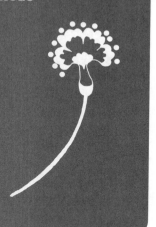

TEN BEST FOODS FOR YOUR NAILS

1. *Broccoli*
2. *Spinach*
3. *Leafy green vegetables*
4. *Brewer's yeast*
5. *Apricots*
6. *Oily fish*
7. *Nuts and seeds*
8. *Tomatoes*
9. *Pulses*
10. *Seaweed and algae such as spirulina*

It's easy to notice that oily fish, dark leafy green vegetables, whole grains, and dairy products contain most hair-friendly vitamins. Base your diet around these foods if you want to improve the condition of your hair naturally.

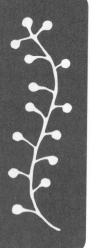

TOP TEN OPTIONS FOR BREAKFAST

1. *Oatmeal with honey, topped with raisins, nuts, and seeds*
2. *Fresh fruit like apples, oranges, bananas, grapes, berries, peaches, plums, nectarines, and pineapple*
3. *½ cup cottage cheese with ½ cup chopped fresh or dried fruit*
4. *½ whole grain bagel topped with ½ tablespoon light cream cheese or natural fruit jam or jelly*

5. *Bircher muesli: oatmeal soaked overnight in plain water. In the morning, add a tablespoon of light cream cheese and dried and fresh fruit*
6. *Fruit and vegetable smoothie: combine any fruit, berries, or vegetables in a blender with ice cubes and some milk or soy drink and blend until smooth*
7. *Crusty bread slices topped with wedges of tomato with celery sticks*
8. *Soft-boiled eggs, omelet, or eggs Benedict*
9. *Yogurt*
10. *Energy bars (for those who are desperately late for work or school). Make sure your energy bar is sweetened with honey, maple, or agave syrup and not sugar. Some of the better energy bars are made by Greens Plus, Now, and BumbleBar. Making your own energy bar is surprisingly easy and satisfying (and economical too). Here's a simple technique that can be modified according to your preferences and availability of ingredients:*

Ingredients

Grains: Feel free to combine your favorite cereals such as rolled oats, toasted wheat germ, rice, or quinoa flakes (mix and match to fill 2 cups).

Fruit: Mix and match any dried fruit such as dried apricots, raisins, and pitted dried dates to fill 1 cup.

Nuts and seeds: Mix and match seeds and nuts as long as they are unsalted and not covered in sugar.

Sweeteners (optional): 1/4 cup honey, maple, or agave syrup.

Spices (optional): a dash of cinnamon, a few drops of pure vanilla extract.

> **Method**
>
> Combine all ingredients in a food processor and pulse until the mixture is uniformly blended. Now spread the mixture evenly in a prepared pan and bake it in a 350° F oven for approximately twenty minutes.

GOING ORGANIC FOR GLOWING SKIN

Once only in the realm of the most dedicated wellness junkie, organic foods are becoming increasingly popular, with every major grocery chain stocking organic foods, and a few even launching their own organic lines. It's hard to argue the main benefit: foods with fewer pesticides are better for my body and for the environment too.

I grew up in Soviet Russia, where families routinely stocked sacks of potatoes, cabbages, onions, pickled cucumbers, tomatoes, and watermelons, and kept apples fresh during the winter in wood chips. Every autumn, my mother would pasteurize a hundred liters of tomato juice, and can countless homemade preserves and jams for the winter ahead, as there would be literally nothing else to eat. Pig heads (yes, complete with eyes and ears, to our naïve amusement) were the only meat available in grocery stores, so naturally, we didn't feast on meat three times a day. Sausages, chicken, and decent bacon were a luxury. So were oranges and bananas. Schoolchildren were sent off to the tomato fields to collect tomatoes or sort corn by hand. I certainly do not want to romanticize that way of life because heaven knows there's nothing romantic about waiting in a queue for hours to be able to buy a frozen, emaciated chicken and turn it into a feast for six using only onions and garlic. But we all understood that you don't need a lot to eat healthily (my mother survived on bland porridge on bad days and had a waist twice smaller than mine today), we were forced to live nearly vegetarian (which is good for your overall health), and we rarely suffered from food allergies or obesity (and I have thankfully passed allergy-free genes to my daughter).

Not many of us have to grow our own foods these days. We expect an endless supply of food all year round even if it means that our little luxuries such as strawberries in January or mangoes in February must come from faraway lands, resulting in greater use of fossil fuels. This side of organic food business doesn't resonate with me: most often, people who crave organic blueberries from Chile in December are ones for whom organic is a trend, not the way of healthy eating. To me, eating organic means supporting local farmers, preserving the quality of our soil and water, and reducing the costs of keeping us healthy and youthful.

The exposure to pesticides is perhaps the main reason to switch to organic fruit and vegetables. Conventionally grown foods are eight to eleven times more likely to contain multiple pesticide residues than organic food. Even if a certain fruit or vegetable, especially those with thicker skin, such as avocado, are generally lower in pesticides, the long-term effects of exposure to multiple pesticides poses a health risk to which many consumers aren't willing to expose themselves or their children. Pesticides are linked with cancer of brain, breast, stomach, prostate, and testicles. Grape farmers and vineyard workers in France have higher rates of brain cancer due to constant exposure to pesticides used in growing grapes for wine production. Childhood leukemia,[78] reduced fertility,[79] thyroid[80] and pituitary disorders,[81] lowered immunity,[82] autism,[83] and attention deficit disorder[84] in children are all linked to high levels of pesticides in the conventional food eaten on daily basis. In addition to pesticides, health risks of irradiated and genetically modified foods containing antibiotics and growth hormones are still largely unknown.

Still, organic products can never be completely free from pesticides. In a world where persistent toxic chemicals pollute the oceans and DDT has been found in Antarctic snow, toxic compounds from the atmosphere, soil, groundwater, and other sources may be beyond the control of the farmer. Instead of conventional, highly toxic, and often carcinogenic pesticides, organic farmers use natural pesticides, such as sulfur, copper, and pyrethrins. They are used sparingly and readily break down in the environment. They also use birds and other insect predators instead of chemical fertilizers, and take advantage of compost and beneficial soil microorganisms. In this way, organic farming makes us and the planet healthier.

Nutritionally, organic fruit and vegetables give you more goodness bang for your buck. Recent studies show that in addition to containing fewer toxic pesticides, organically grown foods provide more vitamins and essential minerals than their conventionally grown counterparts. Organic crops show higher levels of vitamin C,[85] minerals, and antioxidants.[86] Organically raised animals are fed a certified organic diet and never given growth hormones or antibiotics. Plums, peaches, pears, and potatoes have all tested for greater concentrations of nutrients, and animals that ate organic foods showed better growth and reproduction. Studies are now determining whether organically grown food will produce better long-term health in humans too.

Of course, there's also a budget factor. At the first glance, organic apples, carrots, cereals, and meats are more expensive. Of course, using fewer pesticides means more hand-weeding, making labor costs higher, and organic fertilizers and compost are more expensive than chemical brew used in conventional agriculture. But when we buy seemingly affordable, conventionally grown foods, we don't take into account hidden costs of eating chicken squeezed into tiny battery cages and fed fertilizer-soaked corn. All conventional food manufacturers must compensate for contaminated water supplies, toxic waste transportation, not to mention medical bills from farm workers who have paid with their health for "affordable" meals on our table. Researchers put the annual cost of environmental damage caused by industrial farming in the United States at \$34.7 billion.[87] If all these expenses were included in the price of conventionally produced food, it would cost more than organic food.

If you make one dietary change to achieve glowing skin for many years to come, make it this: buy organic whenever you can.

Chapter Four Quick Tips
Nutritional Do's for Glowing Skin

1. Eat more fruits and vegetables. They are full of antioxidants, vitamins, minerals, and fiber. Colorful fruits and vegetables provide more antioxidants than pale-colored ones. **Eat at least two different vegetables with lunch and dinner every day.**
2. **Drink more water, diluted juices, and green tea.** Eat lots of water-rich fruits and vegetables, which are a better source of hydration as the water in plant cells is better absorbed by the body.
3. To maintain collagen and elastin levels, **consume good-quality protein from organic or ethically farmed meat, oily fish, beans, nuts, legumes, and soy products.**
4. **Eat fish twice a week.** Choose smaller fish varieties and avoid farmed fish.
5. **Add healthy oils** rich in anti-inflammatory omega-6 essential fatty acids to your diet and eliminate all processed fats and oils from your meals.
6. **Eat more fiber** in the form of oatmeal, oat bran, dried beans, peas, carrots, broccoli, artichokes, apples, oranges, grapefruits, and whole grains. You can also add bran flakes to any ground meat or vegetable stew recipe.

7. **Cut down on sugar**, which speeds up skin aging and

contributes to weight gain. Replace sugar with stevia or honey and gradually "teach" your taste buds to enjoy less sweet desserts. Replace simple carbs with complex carbs.

8. **Eliminate trans-fats, artificial dyes, synthetic spices, and preservatives** from your foods.
9. **Use spices, fresh herbs, and garlic** generously to add vitamins, minerals, and antioxidants to your meals.
10. **Go organic.** If organic dairy, eggs, or meats are not available, choose free-range options.

Nutritional Don'ts that Ruin Your Natural Beauty

1. **Don't eat heavily processed foods** that are "enriched" with stabilizers, preservatives, and other synthetic junk.
2. **Don't skip meals**, especially breakfast.
3. **Don't eat fried foods.** Bake, broil, or grill foods and make sure your meats do not burn.
4. **Don't clean your plate just to be polite.** Eat only as much as you want. Do not eat leftovers after your kids are finished with their food.
5. **Don't crash diet**: not all of the newest diet crazes will produce sustainable weight loss results, and many diets can actually damage your health and good looks.
6. **Don't buy food in tins and cans**: the plastic lining of cans leaches dangerous phthalates into your food. Opt for glass packaging. Purchase dried legumes, and soak overnight before cooking.
7. **Don't use hydrogenated fats in cooking.**

Hydrogenated fats may increase free radicals in the body. Olive oil or butter is a better choice than margarine.

8. **Don't consume foods and beverages that are overloaded with sugar.** And don't make the mistake of thinking that diet drinks are healthier for you. Artificial sweeteners that are used in diet beverages are known to disrupt your health even more than sugar does.

9. Don't shop on an empty stomach. Set some time aside to plan your meals for the week ahead. Shop at farmers markets and food co-ops, where you can get fresh, local foods.

10. Don't get discouraged. **Be kind to yourself.** Eating healthy will not become your habit for life if you look at it as a burden.

FIVE

Become a Natural Beauty

You already know that to take care of your skin in a holistic way, you must take good care of your whole body. Glowing skin begins on your pillow, on your plate, and in a glass of water or a cup of green tea. As you now know how to treat your skin and hair from the inside out, let's learn how to nourish our beauty from the outside as well.

Long considered an impermeable barrier, our skin is now perceived as a doorway for many chemicals, good and bad. Chemicals with large molecule size cannot be absorbed, but smaller molecules can penetrate the body without any difficulties.[88] Medical science has developed new drugs delivered through the skin directly to the circulation. There are many drugs marketed as transdermal patches, for example, scopolamine (for motion sickness), nicotine (smoking cessation), and estradiol (estrogen deficiency). Scientists believe that skin itself—and especially the outermost layer, the stratum corneum—can play the role of a reservoir for chemicals.[89] In a recent study, Swiss scientists found that even without use of penetration enhancers, human skin absorbs up to 10 percent of all toxins applied to its surface.[90] Another study from 2007 discovered that some chemicals are better able to penetrate the skin; for example, up to 60 percent of parabens applied to the skin surface were found in the epidermis after eight hours.[91]

It is important to choose cosmetic products with the same care with which we choose our food. This chapter explains the two basic concepts of holistic beauty: "Less is more," and "Skincare is food for the skin." To begin our journey into holistic beauty, let's first learn its most important principles.

10 COMMANDMENTS OF WHOLE BEAUTY

The words "natural" and "organic" have become so ubiquitous on product labels, we nearly forget that not all products are created equal. We have to watch out for false claims and loud promises with extra vigilance. As you adopt a holistic approach to beauty, it's time to subject your beauty routine to more scrutiny and to question whether you actually need all those primers, polishes, and potions.

Holistic Beauty Commandment 1: Always check the label
As someone who spent many years trying every skincare product on the market and is now blending natural ingredients for a living and for fun, I can admit: skincare today *is* rocket science, with some of the worst ingredients better off belonging to the rocket fuel tank rather than to our skin. Of course you can continue trusting clever marketers who would have you believe that all their potions and cleansers are good enough to eat, or you can stop falling prey to false claims and take matters in your own hands. There's no way around it: always read the label. If it involves buying a magnifying glass, buy the magnifying glass. Do you research your options when you purchase flights or car insurance? Your skin deserves the same amount of effort.

First, see which proportion of ingredients sounds natural and how far they fall from the beginning of the list. All ingredients in a beauty product are listed in order of the proportion that they are contained in the formula. If there's water in the beginning, then you know this lotion contains lots of water, which isn't necessarily bad. But if alcohol is listed close to the top of the list, this product is bound to be drying and harsh to your skin.

Some ingredients do not need to be used in large quantities to bring good or bad results. You only need a drop of parabens in your body lotion to put you at a higher risk for breast cancer, and you only need a dash of an antiaging peptide to do its magic on your wrinkles.

Do not be put off by strange-sounding eugenols, linalools, and other "-ools" at the end of the list—these are components of essential oils and are usually harmless unless, of course, you are allergic to them. But if you spot some tongue-twisting or clearly synthetic stuff such as ethylhexylglycerine or cyclosyloxane, not to mention any member of the Dirty Dozen list ahead, this product won't do your skin or hair any good.

ORGANIC BEAUTY EXPLAINED

Do you know what a logo means on your organic moisturizer? Here's a quick guide to three most common organic skincare certifiers:

USDA ORGANIC: *This certifying organization has the strictest criteria: it approves only those products that contain 95–100 percent certified organic ingredients. However, be prepared to find lots and lots of alcohol in your lotion or a cleanser, as this is the only preservative approved for the USDA Organic label. To be effective, alcohol should comprise at least 10 percent of the product. Do you really want your baby lotion be similar to your gin and tonic? I don't think so.*

SOIL ASSOCIATION: *The product that carries this stamp contains at least 95 percent organic ingredients. However, the percentage*

> *of organic goodness may be lower if nonorganic ingredients are clearly listed on the label. Excellent and reasonable practice, as most clays, minerals, and vitamins cannot be organic.*
>
> ECOCERT: *France's certifying body is the least strict and permits the use of synthetic fragrances and preservatives in their products. To me, this "organic" logo is meaningless, yet having it on the label is still a good indication of a certain natural commitment from the manufacturer.*

Holistic Beauty Commandment 2: Avoid irritants

You can instantly know there's something wrong with a new beauty product if you notice burning right away, a new rash, redness, or skin flakiness after a few days. When skincare ingredients cause irritation and damage to the protective mantle of the skin, you become susceptible to sun damage, allergies, and even skin infections. Such ingredients include alcohol (especially denatured), menthol, camphor, lemon, and lime in any variation. All members of the Dirty Dozen listed later are potent skin irritants and should be avoided at all costs—not only by those with sensitive skin. Black henna as well as chemicals in conventional hair dyes are very irritating too.

Holistic Beauty Commandment 3: Listen to your skin

Skin types and age-appropriate skincare regimens are things of the past. These days, a twentysomething may have parched skin with visible lines after frequent sunbathing and rigorous acne eradication while some women over fifty have clear, unlined faces and bright eyes. When choosing skincare products, always take into consideration your current skin concerns. If your skin feels dry, go for gentle nourishing oils and natural emollients and humectants such as hyaluronic acid, ceramides, and glycerine. They help retain moisture in your skin by attracting it from the outside air. Because of the increased environmental burden on our bodies, we need antioxidant protection starting at a very young age. To preserve your natural beauty, look for skincare products with natural oils, co-enzyme Q10, green tea, and vitamins A, C, and E as well as soothing plant botanicals. Remember that you cannot supply your skin with collagen and elastin from creams and serums. Instead, at any age, add age-resisting antioxidants to your diet and as carefully selected supplements.

Holistic Beauty Commandment 4: Don't expect miracles overnight
Cosmetic manufacturers want you to believe that you can rub on some potion and wake up to glowing, flawless skin. So we treat the skincare as a magic wand. But in the real world, results are never instant. With a holistic approach to your beauty—that is, practicing stress relief, learning good sleep habits, following healthy diet and using natural skincare—you will aim for sustainable results in the long term. Instead of waiting for the miracle to happen, start making your skin and hair healthier over time, working against the clock. Of course, miracles *do* happen. If you switch from a terrible product to a good one, results are usually seen very quickly (and vice versa). If you apply zit-zapping tea tree oil on an angry blemish, you will wake up to see it "miraculously" decreased in size. If you use an exfoliating peel or a scrub, you will see immediate improvement in the skin texture as dead skin cells are removed. And, of course, a good night's sleep works miracles for your eyes, your skin, and your mood. But if you aim for realistically gradual improvement to your looks, your self-esteem and your general well-being will only benefit.

Holistic Beauty Commandment 5: Remember that price doesn't always equal quality
Just because a cream is expensive doesn't mean it works better. When you compare the ingredient lists of the ten most expensive antiwrinkle creams on the market, you will be surprised to see that most of them contain the very same ingredients. The difference lies in packaging, price of advertising and paid celebrity endorsements, and, of course, the perceived "value" of the brand. Most

cosmetic companies own dozens of brands, both "luxury" and "economy." Do you think that luxury brands are blended in gold-plated vats and hand-poured into crystal tubes by serious professionals in sterile spacesuits, while less expensive creams bubble in dirty buckets and are slapped into plastic tubs with rusty spoons? Well, not exactly. All of them are made in the same factory, in the same blending machines, using ingredients from the same supplier. Some creams and lotions are packed in pump dispensers each costing $10 and covered with layers of boxes and plastic; others are poured in simple plastic bottles costing twenty cents each. There are good and bad products in all price ranges—you need to read ingredients to see which ones work best for you.

An inexpensive rose water will do your skin more good than an expensive toner from a famous brand loaded with preservatives, petrochemicals, and artificial fragrances. Why bother with an expensive anti-blemish toner if plain witch hazel from a health food store is just as good? Why buy expensive eye patches if slices of raw potato remove eye bags and dark circles just as well? I am blessed to have access to amazing oils, hydrosols, and vitamins that we use to make Petite Marie Organics skincare, so instead of buying a new cleanser, I just quickly whip up a new one, throwing in some oils and clays if I feel my skin needs some purifying action, or soothing chamomile and calendula if it's misbehaving. I decant into an old glass bottle and voilà! I am $10 richer. Fussing about famous brand names on the labels of your beauty products is so 1990. All you need is healthy, gentle ingredients for your skin and hair, prepared with minimum preservatives and zero toxic junk. Choose your products based on your skin needs, not to support your status or nourish your ego.

Holistic Beauty Commandment 6: Mix and match as long as you like
Forget the marketing myth saying that you must use cleansers, toners, and moisturizers from one line because they are "designed" to work in synergy. Feel free to use a cleanser from one brand (or

even homemade), mask from another brand, and moisturizer from yet another one—as long as it makes your skin (and wallet) happy. In other words, you should adapt your skincare regimen to your current skin needs.

Holistic Beauty Commandment 7: Play dumb when you hear beauty myths
Myths are created when people are too lazy to look for a reasonable explanation to certain things. One myth is that you need a night cream and a day cream. If your skin is dry, slathering a thick balm at night will not do it any good. Instead, find out why is it dry and act accordingly. Drink more water. Install a humidifier. Toss away that alcohol-laden toner. Add a few drops of oil to your regular moisturizer or massage some oil into your skin at bedtime. Another myth says that people with oily skin should avoid oil in their beauty products because it makes their skin produce more oil. Nonsense! Endocrine glands trigger oil production, not skincare. Our skin has no brains of its own to decide whether it's had enough oil or not. Some oils are quite pore-clogging (cocoa, wheat germ, shea), but thin, "dry" oils such as jojoba, chia, and evening primrose are excellent for oilier skin types.

TOP TEN BEAUTY MYTHS

1. *Vaseline is the number one cure for wrinkles and age spots.*
2. *Toothpaste on blemishes cures them overnight.*
3. *You can shrink your pores.*
4. *Shaving your legs will make your hair grow in thick and coarse.*
5. *Hemorrhoid cream helps eye puffiness vanish.*
6. *Products labeled as hypoallergenic are safe for sensitive skin.*
7. *You can scrub your blackheads away.*
8. *Your skincare should always smell pretty.*
9. *Brushing your hair a hundred times every day makes it shiny.*
10. *Collagen and elastin in skincare help lift the skin.*

Holistic Beauty Commandment 8: Aim for greener packaging
They say that it's the stuff inside the bottle that truly matters. But as you aim to reduce your exposure to chemicals in your skincare, you should pay more attention to the bottle too. PET plastics leach phthalates into your products, especially if there are lots of essential oils or acids in the formula. Aluminum tubes and bottles are usually lined with epoxy resin, which is another mighty source of gender-bending bisphenol-A. Safe plastic for skincare is polypropylene, identified as PP or #5 plastic on the bottom of a container. The safest and most environmentally friendly packaging is glass or cardboard—yes, they can now make cardboard jars for creams and lotions!

Holistic Beauty Commandment 9: Protect your skin from environmental damage
The true source of eternal beauty is smart protection from damaging elements, especially from the sun. But not all SPF is created equal. Synthetic sunscreens often poise more danger than the sun rays they are created to shield against (further on in this book you will learn more about natural sun protection). Instead, use mineral sun blocks made with zinc oxide and to a lesser extent titanium dioxide, as they sit on the skin surface and act as tiny mirrors reflecting dangerous rays of all types instead of penetrating the skin and fighting the enemy on your territory—causing untold damage to the skin and your health in general. Nourish your skin with antioxidants applied topically and consumed with food to protect against chemical vapors, industrial fumes, automobile emissions, volatile organic compounds, free radicals, and other hazardous "additions" in the air.

Holistic Beauty Commandment 10: Protect your skin from inside
The most trustworthy skin and hair health insurance you can buy is not in the jar or a tube but in your refrigerator and in the kitchen cupboard (and, if you are lucky, in your tap). Feeding your skin with glow-promoting nutrients is the most reliable way to smooth, glowing skin and strong, resilient hair. Eating a healthy, wholesome

diet; balancing the stress with meditation and good sleep; and probably taking an antioxidant supplement (or two) will make your skin and hair more beautiful than all the expensive creams and lotions money can buy. You cannot supply your skin with collagen and elastin from creams, and you cannot prevent hair loss with shampoos. True beauty starts inside your body.

THE DIRTY DOZEN

When we book a holiday vacation, choose a health insurance, or buy a car, we spend untold hours online, comparing options and reading reviews. Why don't we approach our beauty products with the same discrimination? Is it only the price difference between a car and a jar of cream that matters? If you add up all those jars, tubes, bottles, and vials that you have purchased over the years, the difference won't be as dramatic. It is estimated that women spend between $2,000 and $20,000 a year on various skin and hair treatments. But when it comes to choosing beauty products, we are so trusting, it is nearly killing us as a result.

Consider this: the sheer amount of synthetic chemicals in use all over the world has increased twentyfold over the last ten years. Today we have over one hundred thousand chemicals in use in different areas of our lives,[92] and less than 5 percent of these chemicals have been thoroughly tested for their long-term impact on human health. Sometimes it takes decades to ban a certain toxin from use in skincare, just as it took nearly forty years for health authorities to admit the health risks of smoking cigarettes.

Even as mounting scientific evidence points at the dangers of a certain ingredients, the cosmetic industry cleverly manipulate these scientific results, calling them "urban legends" or "pseudoscience." Parabens in the breast tissue? Urban legend, says a well-known dermatologist who is busy promoting his own antiaging range. Phthalates found in urine and breast milk? Pseudoscience, says the prominent cancer therapist who is too cautious to admit that nutrition and lifestyle, not just genetics, play an important part in our cancer risk. Lead in lipsticks? Show us the dead bodies, cosmetic regulators say. There's no harm until the harm is done.

The grim reality of the unregulated cosmetic industry leaves us to our own devices. Every day we learn about recalls of toys and clothing contaminated with lead, yet no one has ever recalled red lipsticks where lead exceeds permissible levels. Cosmetics, unlike drugs, are not regulated for safety by the government. It's up to the cosmetic manufacturer to prove the safety of the cosmetic product. That's why you should become a smart natural beauty shopper and learn to read ingredient lists or labels to spot the worst offenders.

Parabens
When absorbed by the skin, these esters of p-hydroxybenzoic acid accumulate in the fat tissue, most notably in the breasts.[93] Samples of breast tissue collected from forty mastectomies for breast cancer in England between 2005 and 2008 found at least one type of parabens in 99 percent of the samples, and all five types of parabens in 60 percent of the samples.[94] These parabens were found in the breast tissue of women of all ages. Even those who said they have never used antiperspirants or deodorants in their underarm area still had parabens in their bodies, which means that our breasts accumulate parabens from all sources. Having lumps of parabens in our bodies is not an urban legend anymore.

What is so harmful about parabens? First of all, parabens are xenoestrogens—chemicals that imitate the action of natural hormones. Xenoestrogens bind to estrogen receptors in the breast tissue and trigger growth. In the body, parabens transform into p-hydroxybenzoic acid, which has a stronger estrogenic response in human breast cancer cells.[95]

Thankfully, there are lots of both conventional and natural cosmetic products made without parabens. The practice of removing these dangerous preservatives is so common, not all manufacturers who avoid parabens advertise it on their labels. Still, if in doubt, look for "paraben-free" on the label. There are so many safe preservatives developed over the last few years, the use of parabens is no longer necessary.

Formaldehyde

Formaldehyde, one of the oldest preservatives used in medicine and skincare, is classified as carcinogenic to humans. Despite this fact, formaldehyde can be found in nail polishes, antiperspirants, makeup, bath products, shampoos, mouthwashes, and deodorants. Popular "Brazilian blow-dry" and similar hair straightening procedures often involve formaldehyde, as do hair-straightening balms, conditioners, and rinses that promise sleek, glossy hair. Formaldehyde is released most actively when you iron or blow-dry your hair using styling products that contain at least one of the following formaldehyde releasers: polyquaterniums, especially quaternium-15; 2-bromo-2-nitropropane-1,3-diol; imidazolidinyl urea; and diazolidinyl urea. Immediate reactions to large amounts of formaldehyde vapors include nausea, headache, and eye irritation that causes tear overflow and a burning sensation in the throat. Long-term effects of formaldehyde exposure include neurotoxicity, genotoxicity, and increased risk of leukemia,[96] as well as brain, liver, nasal, and lung cancers.[97]

Waterproof and crease-proof fabrics, stain-proof carpets, laminated flooring, fiberboard furniture, suede, and nylon often emit formaldehyde.[98] To minimize your exposure, avoid fabrics that underwent heavy treatment and choose solid wood flooring and furniture, if you can. There are many excellent nail polishes made without formaldehyde or toluene (yet another skin and eye irritant).

Avoiding formaldehyde in styling products is a tricky task, but it can be done. To reduce the damage to your health, choose organic and natural hair care products made by John Masters Organics, Lavera, Aubrey Organics, and many other reputable manufacturers (find more suggestions in the Appendix B). Bath and skincare products you use should not contain any formaldehyde releasers and should be either unscented or fragranced with pure essential oils.

Phthalates
Speaking of fragrances, there's nearly impossible to avoid artificial scents these days. Everything we use has some kind of an added scent to it. From household cleaners to candles and even baby toys, smells bombard our senses, often triggering not only positive emotions but also skin rashes, headaches, and teary eyes. Surprise: the irritating compounds in artificial fragrances are not the worst offenders. You cannot smell phthalates, but they do your health as much damage as parabens or formaldehyde. Phthalates are industrial chemicals used as softeners in plastics made of polyvinyl chloride (PVC) and solvents in artificial fragrances. Epidemiological studies link phthalate exposure to the following:

> IN MEN: shorter penis, sperm DNA damage, decreased proportion of healthy sperm, and low sperm concentration.[99]
> IN WOMEN: breast cancer,[100] abnormally early puberty (as early as six years),[101] endometriosis,[102] and hyperprolactinemia.[103]
> IN CHILDREN: attention deficit hyperactivity disorder,[104] low intelligence quotient.[105]
> IN ALL ADULTS: rhinitis,[106] eczema,[107] asthma,[108] thyroid hormone alteration,[109] obesity,[110] and diabetes.[111]

Which beauty products are "richest" in phthalates? According to a 2011 study among women in Mexico, the highest concentration of phthalates in their bodies appeared from use of body lotions, deodorants and antiperspirants, fragrances, antiaging facial creams, and bottled water.[112] Unfortunately, cosmetic manufacturers now focus their efforts on young girls. My five-year-old daughter now wants glittery makeup, nail polish, and an eau de toilette with her favorite kitten or princess on the packaging. I usually win the battle by painting her nails with chemical-free nail polish in a bright pink shade and letting her use my own organic lip glosses and eye shadows. But what about the millions of girls whose parents are not into natural skincare? These girls will be exposed to phthalates, formaldehyde, and artificial colorants so early, and their bodies won't be able to cope with all that chemical rubbish.

Other significant sources of phthalates are baby bottles made of polycarbonate that leach bisphenol A into drinks and food, and canned foods that absorb phthalates from epoxy resin lining tin and aluminum cans. Shower curtains, rubber ducks, PVC furniture and clothes, sex toys, fragrances, MP3 players—phthalates are so ubiquitous, it is impossible to completely avoid them. Here are some steps that you can take to get rid of at least some of the phthalates in your environment:

1. Avoid drinking water, or any other beverage, from a plastic bottle. Buy mineral water in glass bottles if you can. Once you have one large glass bottle, refill it with filtered water or tap, if you are lucky to live in a place where tap water is clean enough to drink unfiltered. Alternatively, carry your water supply in steel canisters but make sure they are not lined with epoxy resin, which can also leach phthalates. Less expensive plastic bottles made from polypropylene (identified as plastic 5 or PP at the bottom) are still a better option than polycarbonate and polyethylene terephthalate (PET) bottles.

2. Do not eat canned food. Choose toothpaste, ointments, and creams packaged in plastic rather than aluminum tubes, which are always lined with phthalate-rich epoxy resin. Steel and aluminum

water bottles must be labeled as BPA (bisphenol A) free. Choose canned tomatoes in glass jars. Tomato juice and oils in foods absorb phthalates most efficiently. Unfortunately, there are no options for BPA-free canned fish. Buy fresh fish, then cook and freeze small portions—it will be much better for your health.

3. Limit your exposure to artificial fragrances. Whenever you sense a synthetic smell of roses, understand that at that very moment phthalates are entering your lungs. Choose unscented laundry detergents and household cleaners. Switch to greener brands such as Seven Seas, which uses essential oils to scent their cleaning products. Better yet, add a few drops of your favorite essential oil to the laundry detergent or the floor cleaner. Instead of a heavily scented phthalate-rich air freshener, use a votive candle or a scented cone that you can buy from most health food stores.

4. Choose nail polish that is marked as phthalate free or BPA free, or at least toluene free. That's a good sign that a manufacturer took care to remove toxic ingredients from its products. Many manufacturers including Revlon, Clinique, and Clarins are now removing toxins from their nail products, but to be absolutely sure, choose polishes from Suncoat or Zoya. You can find more suggestions at the end of this book.

Aluminum

Every morning, as you reach for a stick or a roller with a freshly scented antiperspirant liquid, consider this: at this very moment, you are poisoning your breasts, and your brain.

All antiperspirants on the market rely on aluminum in the form of aluminum chloride, aluminum zirconium, and aluminum chlorohydrate. Even the so-called natural antiperspirants with "mineral salts" appear to contain alum, a mineral salt chemically known as aluminum potassium sulfate. Natural or not, aluminum is still present.

When applied to the skin, aluminum salts dry out sweat by injecting aluminum ions into the cells that line the sweat ducts. When the aluminum ions are drawn into the cells, water flows in; the cells begin to swell, squeezing the ducts closed so that sweat cannot get out. But aluminum stays inside the body.

A potent neurotoxin, aluminum enters our bloodstream in large doses, contributing to two serious diseases: breast cancer and Alzheimer's disease, which is the most common cause of dementia, affecting millions of men and women worldwide. Upon reaching the brain, this metal alters the function of the blood-brain barrier. Scientists have found that plaques in the brains of Alzheimer's disease sufferers contain aluminum.[113]

Every day we rub aluminum-loaded antiperspirant into our underarm areas, where many lymph nodes are located close to the surface of the skin. Numerous studies link breast cancer to long-term use of aluminum-based antiperspirants. Dr. Philippa D. Darby of the University of Reading in the United Kingdom has shown that aluminum salts increase estrogen-related gene expression in human breast cancer cells grown in vitro, which makes aluminum a powerful metalloestrogen.[114] Of course, aluminum is not the main cause of breast cancer and brain diseases. There are many factors involved in the progression of both ailments including lifestyle, diet, and heredity. But wouldn't you avoid one significant factor if you could? I hope you will. And you won't go around smelly and wet. In Chapter Twelve, you will find more about natural alternatives to cancer-causing antiperspirants.

Sodium Laureth Sulfate
One of the harshest detergents ever created by a chemist, this petroleum-derived foaming agent is widely used in shampoos,

skin cleansers, toothpastes, and baby washes. Sodium laureth sulfate (SLS) is a strong irritant and is known to frequently cause allergic dermatitis. Besides the health risks, SLS is not biodegradable and is a considerable poison to waterways and wildlife.

Recent studies have found that sodium laureth sulfate and similar detergents made with ethoxylated compounds may be contaminated with low doses of 1,4-dioxane,[115] a strong toxin and a known human carcinogen. While there are no reliable methods to instantly detect 1,4-dioxane in skincare products unless you are willing to send a sample to a chemist, it would make sense to avoid sodium laureth sulfate as well as other ethoxylated ingredients. You can easily identify them on the product label by letters -*eth* in the name, for example, laur*eth*, myr*eth*, and cet*eth*. There are so many natural cleansing agents available for face and body cleansing, it would be a shame to continue using shampoos or body washes with SLS.

Propylene Glycol

Propylene glycol is one of the most popular cosmetic ingredients. It helps active ingredients penetrate the skin more efficiently; it is an emollient and humectant, helping draw moisture from the air. Originally formulated for the car industry, it is used in baby washes, bubble baths, deodorants, shampoos, hair dyes, and even personal lubricants.

The FDA considers propylene glycol to be "generally recognized as safe" for use in food, cosmetics, and medicines. However, if you have sensitive or acne-prone skin, this ingredient is definitely to be avoided.

Contact allergic dermatitis is the most common side effect of using products containing propylene glycol and similar petrochemicals such as polyethylene glycol (PEG) and ethylene glycol[116]

Irritation and rashes are unpleasant, of course, but there's yet another danger about petrochemicals used in skincare products.

Toxicology studies found that common cosmetic ingredients contain such dangerous substances as ethylene oxide, 1,4-dioxane, polycyclic aromatic compounds, and heavy metals such as lead, iron, cobalt, nickel, cadmium, and arsenic. Despite such concerns, PEG compounds remain commonly used in "natural" cosmetics and personal care products, often disguised by giving plant names to them. For example, a well-known natural deodorant (thankfully, aluminum free) contains more than 50 percent propylene glycol. If you would like to reduce your current personal toxic load, it may make sense to avoid using products containing glycols, especially since so many natural emollients and waxes are available these days.

Hydroquinone
Hydroquinone is used in skin-lightening products to reduce skin color pigment by disrupting the synthesis of melanin. Several surveys and studies including several thousand individuals have shown that regular use of skin-lightening products can have irreversible adverse effects, such as patchy pigmentation, skin atrophy, stretch marks, and delayed wound healing, as well as Cushing's syndrome and eye and kidney damage.[117]

Skin-lightening products with hydroquinone are one of the most dangerous beauty items women are using these days. Because hydroquinone lightens skin by reducing melanin, it simultaneously increases exposure to UVA and UVB rays. This increases skin cancer risks due to UV exposure, in addition to the carcinogenic effects of hydroquinone itself.

Apart from skin damage, hydroquinone is considered highly toxic and carcinogenic even by the most conservative cosmetic authority, the Cosmetic Ingredient Review panel. They approved the use of this bleach in hair dyes and nail products but not in facial skincare.[118]

Back in 1996, the FDA revoked its previous approval of hydroquinone and proposed a ban on all over-the-counter preparations with this chemical. The FDA Carcinogenicity Assessment

Committee stated that hydroquinone is a proven human carcinogen.[119] The US National Library of Medicine lists hydroquinone among serious disruptors of the immune system, and the International Agency for Research on Cancer clearly labels hydroquinone as a carcinogen and mutagen (causing gene mutations leading to cancer).

Despite the scientific evidence, hydroquinone is used in bestselling creams and serums sold worldwide. Safer alternatives to hydroquinone are vitamin C, niacinamide, and arbutin. In the next chapters you will learn about safe and natural ways to boost your skin's clarity.

Denatured Alcohol

To use alcohol in cosmetics, manufacturers must ensure it is a chemical and not an alcoholic beverage. That's why various additives as acetone, methyl ethyl ketone, and denatonium saccharide, the bitterest chemical compound ever known, are added to alcohol, which is then used in conventional toners, cleansers, masks, and moisturizers. Denatonium is an active ingredient in preparations applied to children's nails to prevent nail biting.

To avoid the drying effects of alcohol and toxic effects of denatured alcohol, it is ideal to avoid any alcohol in your skincare products unless it is listed very low in the ingredients list or marked as organic grain or grape alcohol.

Mineral Oil and Petrolatum

These odorless and tasteless liquid hydrocarbons are produced during distillation of gasoline from crude oil. When applied to the skin, mineral oil forms a waterproof film on the surface. Do you think your skin enjoys being wrapped in plastic every day? Needless to say, all vitamins, minerals, and botanicals in the cream are rendered useless because they cannot permeate the mineral oil barrier. Mineral oil blocks the pores and alters skin's natural respiration. With regular use, mineral oil may cause allergic reactions and worsen skin dryness.

Talc

Microscopic talc particles used in cosmetics and baby powders are linked to high risk of lung injury. When inhaled, talc particles stick to lung cells irritating them, blocking airways, and in some cases causing a disease called talcosis. People who work with talc and asbestos often suffer from lung cancer. Along with silica and asbestos, talc particles in home environments are linked to acute respiratory infections in children and chronic obstructive pulmonary disease in women, French scientists have found.[120]

There are even more dangers about talc. Several studies conducted over the past twenty-five years found an association between perineal talc powders and ovarian cancer.[121] Norwegian oncologists believe that talc and asbestos are "ovarian carcinogens."[122] Instead of a talc baby powder consider using cornstarch, rice flour, or powdered lavender and calendula.

Artificial Dyes

Many artificial dyes used in makeup and skincare are strong allergens and even carcinogens. Let's take a look at some of the most frequently used dyes.

FD&C Blue No. 1 (Brilliant Blue 1, E133) is a proven neurotoxin that may induce an allergic reaction, especially if you suffer with asthma, even when used in very small quantities. This dye has been banned from use in food in Austria, Belgium, Denmark, France, Germany, Greece, Italy, Norway, Spain, Sweden, and Switzerland. Still, there is no ban on use of this neurotoxic dye in cosmetic products. This dye can be found in moisturizers, shampoos, and even organic skincare.

FD&C Blue No. 2 (Indigotine, E132) has proven mutagenic and carcinogenic qualities in animal studies.[123] This dye is irritating to skin and eyes. It has been restricted for use in food products but is still allowed for use in cosmetics.

FD&C Green No. 3 (Fast Green, E143) is a toxic dye that is irritating to eyes, skin, and digestive and respiratory tracts. At the moment, FD&C Green No. 3 dye is rarely used in food but found in toothpastes, mouthwashes, deodorants, and even baby skincare products.

FD&C Red No. 40 (Allura Red, E129) is a proven neurotoxin. Several studies have found that FD&C Red No. 40 as well as other azo dyes increased levels of hyperactivity and attention deficit hyperactivity disorder in children consuming sweets, desserts, and drinks containing these dyes. In skincare, this dye is added to body products, moisturizers, and eye creams as well as self-tanning products.

FD&C Red No. 3 (Erythrosine, E127) is a proven carcinogen with numerous studies proving its mutagenic activity. For example, a May 2011 study from the University of Miami found that "erythrosine . . . showed cellular effects including clear cytotoxic effects."[124] This pink dye is very appealing to children. Perhaps for this reason it can be found in children's sunscreen and toothpastes.

FD&C Yellow No. 5 (Tartrazine) is a proven neurotoxin linked to anxiety, migraines, clinical depression, and ADHD in children. It damages the lining of the stomach and alters the healthy function of kidneys. Tartrazine consumption is linked to itching, general weakness, the feeling of suffocation, purple skin patches, and sleep disturbance. People with asthma and aspirin intolerance are especially prone to allergic reactions to tartrazine. As of this writing tartrazine has not been banned in the United States or the European Union although many countries have called for a voluntary ban of this toxic colorant.

FD&C Yellow No. 6 (Sunset Yellow) is a neurotoxin linked to anxiety, migraines, depression, and hyperactivity in children. Sunset Yellow itself may cause allergic reactions with various symptoms, including stomach upset, diarrhea, vomiting, nettle rash (also known as urticaria), and swelling of the skin. Many countries including the United Kingdom proposed a voluntarily ban. At the same time, this synthetic colorant is widely used in the United States and Canada in food, shampoos, moisturizers, and pregnancy and baby products.

This list is by no means exhaustive. Please check your skincare and cosmetic products for the presence of any toxic colorants that may give you allergies, skin rashes, and dermatitis. Besides making your skin look less than pretty, they also directly affect your health and undermine your immune system, which can result in a variety of skin conditions.

We have all ingested our share of parabens, mineral oil, formaldehyde, hydroquinone, and phthalates, to name just a few offenders. Chronic diseases require decades of toxic lifestyle to take hold. Hundreds of women walk around with breast cancer that started in their teens but may not progress until these women reach menopause. But there's no need to despair. The human body is an amazing, complex system with incredible powers of self-regeneration. All it needs is a little helping hand. Let us try to mend the damage. In the next chapter you will learn about natural ways to make you more beautiful without sacrificing your health.

FOXY FIVE: THE GOOD GUYS IN YOUR SKINCARE

As you become more literate in cosmetic ingredient lingo, you will notice that some ingredients, often strange and chemical sounding, occupy the beginning of the list of ingredients. This means that these ingredients comprise up to 90 percent of the product. So it's worth knowing the good guys that do the majority of the skin protection, cleansing, and repairing.

1. *Water. It can be purified, demineralized, or mineral, but water is the most abundant ingredient in beauty products, except for face and beauty oils. In my own experience, magnesium-rich water such as Vichy and Volvic as well as selenium-rich water in La*

Roche-Posay products is most beneficial for the skin. I have concerns about formulations of conventional products with mineral water, as most of them contain preservatives and artificial fragrances. You are much better off buying Vichy or La Roche-Posay water in a spray bottle to use as a toner or a facial mist.

2. *Natural oils and butters.* They lock the moisture in the skin, keep it pliable, and protect skin cell membranes from damage. Certain plant oils, such as evening primrose, rosehip, and olive oils, have antioxidant and anti-inflammatory abilities as well. Beware of comedogenic oils such as cocoa and wheat germ. They can be used in body products but keep them away from facial skin.

3. *Humectants.* These ingredients help to moisturize the skin by attracting the moisture from outside and retaining it inside the skin. Thanks to humectants, our skin remains soft and flexible. Look for ingredients such as glycerine, sugars (mannitol, fructose), and hyaluronic acid, the queen bee of humectants.

4. *Vitamins.* The most beneficial topical vitamin for the skin is vitamin E, which comes in the form of tocopherol acetate (synthetic) or tocotrienols (natural). Vitamin C contained in many products is rendered useless if the shelf life of a product is longer than fourteen days; look for dry vitamin C such as magnesium ascorbyl phosphate, which should be added to creams or serums. You can also buy ester-C (oil-soluble vitamin C) in pharmacies and use it topically as a skin serum. Vitamins C and E work in synergy, so look for both vitamins in the list of ingredients.

5. *Antioxidants.* Beta-carotene, pomegranate, green tea, resveratrol, pycnogenol, lycopene, and quercetin are often added to organic and natural beauty products. Not only do they protect your skin from premature aging, they also ward off immediate dangers such as sunburn and blotchiness.

Chapter Five Quick Tips

1. **Always read the ingredients lists on new beauty products**. If you are dedicated to certain natural products, make sure to check their ingredients once in a while. The higher the ingredient is on the list, the greater proportion it contributes to the product. But, even if a tongue-twisting chemical is listed at the end of the list, still take heed: even if there's only 1 percent of a toxic ingredient per 5 oz. (150 ml) bottle of a body lotion, this is still 1.5 mL of pure, undiluted toxin than you will rub into your skin. Avoid irritants in your beauty products such as alcohol, harsh essential oils, petrochemical emulsifiers, and penetration enhancers. If you are prone to allergies, choose the product with the fewest ingredients.

2. Have reasonable expectations and **do not pay premium for beauty products that promise miracles overnight.**

3. **Mix and match cleansers, toners, and moisturizers as you like**, as long as your skin feels happy about your combinations.

4. Choose biodegradable packaging that does not leach phthalates or other plastic compounds into your products. **Avoid aluminum containers that are lined with epoxy resin and PET bottles that can leach phthalates** in your beauty products.

5. **Avoid cosmetics and hair care that contain one or more of the ingredients listed in the Dirty Dozen.** Any ingredient that has a tongue-twisting chemical name is probably not good for your skin.

SIX

Beautiful Face

True beauty begins with glowing skin. When blemish free, firm, and even toned, our skin tells the outside world about our inner peace and well-being. Achieving beautiful skin and lustrous, strong hair is easier than you think. And it's also a perfectly natural process. The mainstream cosmetic industry can make things look too complicated when in fact all you need is a simple regime that fits your lifestyle, and a few natural products that your skin loves. Good news: the best things you can do for your skin are also absolutely free. Positive attitude, stress relief, and beauty sleep cost nothing yet make dramatic difference to your skin and hair condition. In this chapter you will learn how to take care of your skin, body, and hair in the most natural, holistic way.

MAKE YOUR OWN BEAUTY PRODUCTS

Why would you use expensive but inefficient products overloaded with preservatives, petrochemicals, and hormone-disrupting fragrances that cause irritation, dryness, premature aging, and possibly put you at greater risk for skin cancer, when there is a whole world of inexpensive, safe, and all-natural skincare waiting right there, in the refrigerator, on your kitchen shelves, at the fresh produce department in the grocery store, or on counter of the local farmer's market? Why pay a hefty premium for a moisturizer that costs less than a dollar to prepare at home?

Making your own beauty products is not only cost-effective; it's more ethical, eco-friendly, and skin-friendly too. When your make your own cleanser, toner, or mask, you do not use any fillers such as silicone or water to lower costs. Unless you plan to sell your homemade beauty creations, you don't need any synthetic preservatives—to stay on the safe side, you can add some natural germ-busting vitamin E or rosemary essential oil to your cream so that it's shelf life will be extended by a few months. You are in absolute control of which ingredients to use and which ones to skip. And, of course, you don't need to torture any rabbits or mice to make sure your homemade concoctions are safe to use. If a mask gives you a tingle, rinse it off and discard it. No expensive packaging wasted or synthetic fragrance washed down the drain!

For me, the sheer practicality of making my own cleansers, scrubs, and masks at home was a deciding factor. When you look at the ingredients of your average facial toner in a pretty bottle sold in a department store, you can notice that water, propylene glycol, and glycerine make up the bulk of the product, and perhaps one or two plant hydrosols tucked between silicones and preservatives. Why would you pay $20 for a brew that is more suitable for window cleaning if you can pay four times less for a large bottle of rose water, add a teaspoon glycerine, perhaps a pinch of vitamin C, and the contents of an olive leaf extract capsule for a good measure? If feeling very adventurous, you can enrich your toner with a teaspoon of hyaluronic acid and a few drops of a good antioxidant (check out the list of suppliers for small-scale cosmetic DIY enthusiasts at the end of this book).

Maybe your skin toner would not look as pristine and crystal clear as the store-bought version. The bottle may be quite simple too, with a handwritten label (if any). Maybe there would be some odd bits floating inside and you would need to shake it well before each use. But you can rest assured knowing that everything inside the bottle is safe, natural, and even good enough to eat. And spending five minutes of your precious time, you would have saved at least $18, not to mention the plastic junk that didn't end up in a landfill. A small savings, but it adds up to a substantial amount by the end of the year. Simply by not buying commercially made skincare, I saved nearly $500 and up to twenty pounds of plastic and cardboard over the course of one year.

GETTING CLEAN

How well do you cleanse? If you are like me ten years ago, you spread a dollop of some cleansing gel or a lotion around your face, rub-rub-rub, splash with water, and think it's done. Not quite so.

Imagine this: As you wander through your day, your body remains cozy and relatively clean underclothing. Your scalp is protected by the hair. But your face is always out there, covered by layers of makeup or, if you skip makeup and sun protection, meeting environmental aggressors naked and fragile. Imagine the amount of dirt—all that soot, smoke and gasoline residue, makeup, stale sebum, dry sweat, dead bacteria—piling up on your face by the end of the day. All you need to do to get rid of that is two minutes with a good cleanser. Yes, just two minutes. Set your clock.

Cleansing is the most important facial beauty ritual, and it's very easy to do it right. Just foaming and rinsing isn't enough to remove all that environmental grime and slime. The secret to good cleansing is to use two types of a cleanser one after another, or one cleanser, but twice. The first time will remove makeup and surface dirt; the second time gets deep into the pores to remove any sebum buildup and dead skin cells.

What kind of cleanser do you need? This completely depends on your current skin condition, not on your self-diagnosed skin type, age, or ethnicity. Skin feels tight after being rinsed with plain water? Stick to creamy, milky cleansing lotions or cleansing balms. Skin looks shiny and dripping oil by midday? You will need a purifying cleanser to prevent any acne outbreaks and to remove any junk that sticks more eagerly to excess sebum. Your sensitive skin will benefit from water-thin cleansing oil that turns into milk when water is added. Feel free to mix and match your cleansers depending on your makeup usage. In the morning, you may not need a thorough cleanse at all—just a quick splash of tepid water and a swipe of cotton wool drenched in rosewater.

Here's a step-by-step technique of a two-minute cleanse that you should do every evening, starting today:

First, remove all hair from your face and cleanse your hands. Always start with perfectly clean hands, even if you plan to use a muslin cloth with your cleanser.

Take a fingertip-size amount of your favorite cleanser (gel, cream, lotion, or balm). If you want to cleanse really well, use the creamy, oil-based cleanser first or even cleansing oil—these are good for all skin types, not just for dry skins. Massage the cleanser into your face starting at the chin where it meets the neck and up toward the hairline at the forehead. Massage well and gently while counting to sixty. Rinse off with tepid water.

If you are using the same cleanser, take a smaller amount and repeat the procedure. If you are a cleansing perfectionist, your second cleanse should be a foaming gel or even an exfoliating cleanser with smooth particles of jojoba wax, or natural acids derived from grains and fruits. This cleanser will go deeper into your pores and remove any potential threats for acne, uneven pigmentation, or early wrinkles. Another excellent exfoliating tool is muslin cloth, which you can rub into your skin with your fingertips and adjust the pressure as necessary. Again, massage to the count of sixty, rinse, and pat face dry.

You can easily make your own cleansing lotions and face washes at home using commonly available ingredients. You can add your own bells and whistles to these very simple recipes. For example, you can add vitamins C and E, antioxidants, green tea extract, or clays to the mix—but you can just as well keep things simple. Here are some ideas to get you going:

Yogurt and lemon face rinse: Combine 1 teaspoon plain yogurt with a few drops of fresh lemon juice for an exfoliating cleanser that won't scrub your skin.

Olive oil cleansing gel: Add ½ cup olive oil (or any other oil of your choice) to 100 mL (3.3 fl. oz.) natural liquid soap (castile soap is the best). Shake gently and use generously to cleanse dry skin.

Aloe vera cleansing milk: Combine 3 tablespoons Aloe vera gel with 1 cup of soy milk. Use to remove makeup and cleanse your sensitive skin.

Citrus cleanser: Add 2–3 tablespoons of grapefruit juice to 1 cup of olive oil and shake well as you would while preparing salad dressing. Use daily to remove all traces of makeup, even waterproof types.

Cleansing powder: Combine 2 tablespoons wheat germ, 2 tablespoons polenta or rice grains, and 1 tablespoon corn or gram flour. Keep in a tightly closed jar. To cleanse your skin, take 1 teaspoonful of the mixture, add some water to create a paste and massage gently into your skin. Rinse and pat skin dry.

Egg and milk cleanser: Combine 1 egg and 1 cup of whole milk. Whisk thoroughly until fully blended. Transfer into a clean bottle. Use with a washcloth or a cotton wool to gently cleanse your dry skin. If you are vegetarian, you can use any plant-derived "milk" such as almond or soy drink and some vegetable shortening instead of an egg.

Cleansing Clays

Soft clays such as rhassoul mud are a godsend for people with very sensitive skin who cannot tolerate even cleansing milks, not to mention conventional foaming cleansers. When mixed with water, clays form a colloidal, milk-like substance that absorbs any impurities and penetrates the pores without damaging the skin's protective acid and oil barrier. Here's how you can cleanse your skin with clay:

1. Disperse 1 tablespoon of clay of your choice (I recommend bentonite, Fuller's Earth, or rhassoul mud) in 100 mL (3.3 fl. oz.) water.
2. Add ½ teaspoon psyllium husks, a common fiber supplement, to the mix. Stir well.
3. Decant to a bottle with a wide neck. You can store the blend in the refrigerator for two weeks.

To cleanse your skin, shake the bottle well. The liquid should be the consistency of soft custard. Pour a blob of the mixture into your palm and use as a regular cleanser to massage your skin. Rinse and pat face dry.

Follow the double-cleansing procedure with a toner, which can be a plant hydrosol such as rose or orange water or even a spritz of mineral water.

Using a Face Toner

Toner is a wonderful addition to your skincare routine. Not only does it remove all traces of the cleanser and soften the skin, it also leaves a weightless layer of essential oils, vitamins, and minerals on the skin's surface. In fact, face toner is the most effective leave-on treatment that will never clog your pores or leave a shiny residue.

Toners made from mineral water and floral waters, also known as hydrosols or steam distillates, are easy to make, yet are much better for your skin than conventional formulas, which are rarely anything other than a mix of alcohol, petrochemicals, and preservatives. You can mix and match plant hydrosols or add a teaspoon of apple cider vinegar, a few drops of tinctures, or even a pinch of clay to make your own blends for your current skin condition.

Organic fruit juices (100 percent), fresh milk, and plant-derived drinks such as soy and almond "milks," make great toners. Apply them straight from the container with a cotton pad. Here are some easy homemade toner recipes that take just minutes to prepare:

> **Grapefruit astringent for oily skin:** Combine ½ cup grapefruit juice with ½ cup witch hazel. Keep tightly closed. Apply with a cotton pad—do not mist as the mixture will sting your eyes.
>
> **Rose water mist:** Combine 1 cup rose water with 1 teaspoon witch hazel and 1 teaspoon glycerine or honey. Place in a bottle with a spray top. Shake well to completely blend the ingredients.
>
> **Apple cider vinegar pore cleanser:** Add 2–3 teaspoons apple cider vinegar to 1 cup of green tea. Apply with a cotton pad—do not mist because it will sting your eyes.
>
> **Cooling skin mist:** Prepare 1 cup peppermint tea and 1 cup green tea, and then combine in a bottle with a spray top. Keep in a refrigerator for a refreshing mist after a hot summer day. This simple recipe works wonders on sun-drenched complexion and helps soothe sunburns.
>
> **Cucumber skin rejuvenator:** Extract juice from 1

cucumber either using a juicer or simply by processing the chopped cucumber and then squeezing out the juice from the pulp. Combine with witch hazel for a pore-tightening and cooling drink of moisture for your skin.

Herbal ice cubes: Chop fresh dill, parsley, rosemary, mint, or any other herbs you may have in your garden or on the windowsill and place them in a bowl. Pour some boiling water on top of the herbs and allow to sit until completely cooled (cover the bowl with a saucer to prevent precious essential oils from evaporating). Transfer the herbal water with bits of herbs into ice cube trays and freeze. Use ice cubes to wipe your face after cleansing.

Chamomile skin lightener: Prepare a cup of chamomile tea and add a pinch of vitamin C. Chamomile has a mild brightening effect on your complexion. Shake well and use with a cotton pad. Store this toner in a refrigerator.

Red wine antiaging toner: Add 2–3 teaspoons of good quality red wine (cabernet variety is the best) to 1 cup of rose water or any other steam distillate you prefer. Use with a cotton pad or as a skin mist.

Exfoliate to Rejuvenate

Exfoliating at least twice a week is essential for a glowing, clear complexion, but many conventional scrubs contain harsh exfoliating grains that can leave your skin dry, red, and irritated. If you scrub your face too vigorously, you will remove the protective barrier leaving your skin vulnerable to environmental aggressors including UV rays.

Making your own facial scrub or peel is very easy. I am sure you already own lots of things that can be used in your own scrub, including breakfast cereals, baking soda, fine sea salt, fine sugar, salt, fine polenta, fine oatmeal, rice grains, and even ground coffee. You can make a super-easy scrub with one or more of these ingredients by adding some water or plant hydrosol to a teaspoon of the exfoliating granules of your choice.

Make sure to gently massage your exfoliating cream into your skin, concentrating on the areas where dead skin cells tend to build up: around your nose, chin, and the sides of your face. Do not forget the upper neck area. Unlike harsh conventional scrubs, gentle homemade solutions mildly remove only very superficial skin cells without causing micro-tears.

Here are basic skin scrubs that you can customize to your liking with essential oils and vitamins C and E, if desired.

> **Sugar and yogurt scrub:** Combine 1 teaspoon very fine sugar or even castor sugar with 1 teaspoon yogurt and stir well to mix completely. This scrub is suitable for all skin types.
>
> **Almond and sour cream scrub:** Combine a teaspoon of ground almonds with a teaspoon of sour cream. This scrub is excellent for dry skin.
>
> **Green tea scrub:** Empty the contents of one sachet of green tea or chai drink and add a little boiling water. Allow to cool and use to exfoliate your skin with a paste that is bursting with antioxidants.
>
> **Honey and oatmeal face rub:** Combine ½ cup warm water with 2 tablespoons of oatmeal and 1 teaspoon honey. To use, gently massage your skin with a dollop of the cleanser. You can store the unused product in the refrigerator. This cleanser is especially suitable for people with sensitive skin who cannot tolerate foaming cleansers.

If you have uneven skin texture with large pores and possibly some discolorations from past blemishes and too much sun exposure, facial peels will help achieve a smoother, more even complexion and possibly lighten discolorations. Unlike the scrub that physically removes the top layer of dead skin cells, peels dissolve dead skin cells and also deliver brightening and lightening ingredients deeper into the epidermis.

Please remember that even natural skin peels made with fruit acids can leave your skin liable to sun damage. That's why if you decide to brighten things up a little using alpha- or beta-hydroxy acids in a ready-made facial peel, or to prepare a peeling solution of your own, make sure to protect your skin with a natural sun block with zinc oxide.

> **Lemon skin peel:** Add 1 teaspoon fresh lemon juice to 1 tablespoon of fruit jelly and stir well. Apply to cleansed skin and allow to sit for ten to twelve minutes, then rinse and pat skin dry.
>
> **Apple skin peel:** Add 1 teaspoon apple cider vinegar to 1 tablespoon applesauce. If the paste is too runny, add a little corn flour (cornstarch) to make it easier to apply. Spread over your cleansed skin and allow to sit for ten to fifteen minutes, and then rinse with cool water and pat face dry.
>
> **Potato skin brightener:** Unlike peels, this recipe lightens your skin thanks to the enzyme catecholase in the raw potato, which normalizes the production of skin pigment melanin. Grate 1 raw potato and squeeze the juice from the pulp. Add a little corn or potato starch to create a paste and apply over your cleansed face. Allow to sit for ten to fifteen minutes, rinse with tepid water, and pat face dry.

Moisturizing and Protecting

A good moisturizer can't be too rich or too thin. The skin is in a constant process of renewal, and when wrapped in a protective blanket of a moisturizer, skin can recuperate from dryness and improve its resilience. Ideally, you should moisturise twice a day, in the morning and in the evening. However, your morning moisturizer can double as a sunscreen, and your evening moisturizer can be a light facial oil or an intensive treatment serum. You can also hydrate your skin throughout the day—just a mist of a cooling toner or mineral water can do wonders to rejuvenate tired skin.

Every moisturizer is a mix of ingredients that form a barrier on the skin to slow down the evaporation of water and help skin heal and recuperate: humectants, which act as moisture magnets; and emollients, which add lubrication and help the skin look smoother. It's a myth that a moisturizer "sinks in" the skin, feeding it moisture. Any water in its formula evaporates off the skin surface within minutes after application. Most often, moisturizers contain quite a lot of alcohol which helps evaporate the water even more quickly. Unless the moisturizer contains ingredients that attract the water from outside, it does not supply any water to your skin. All it does is lock the skin's natural moisture inside with oil, plant wax, or beeswax. In conventional moisturizers, paraffin and mineral oil work to lock the moisture inside the skin.

To soften the skin, a moisturizer must contain a natural emollient, which could be a plant-derived silicone from mushrooms or squalane from olives. To attract the moisture from outside, nothing beats glycerine or various sugars such as maltitol or sorbitol. Throw in some mighty antioxidants such as oil-soluble vitamin C called L-ascorbic acid, vitamin E (natural tocopherols and tocotrienols), green tea extract, alpha lipoic acid, coenzyme Q10, or lycopene, and your moisturizer will become a powerful tool to help your skin retain its youthful and blemish-free looks.

The most important function of a moisturizer is maintaining your skin's own protective barrier. Young skin has a strong protective barrier thanks to its thicker epidermis, healthier sebum composition, denser collagen fibers, and better circulation in the skin. As we age, our skin loses its vitality and its protective barrier becomes less efficient. Pollution, smoking, poor diet, too much sun exposure, and hormonal fluctuations mean more wear and tear on the protective barrier. As a result, our skin loses its ability to hold its own moisturizer, water. When water evaporates more easily, our skin looks and feels tight and dry, possibly even flaky and cracking. That's when the moisturizer should step in.

One of the most important ingredients in your moisturizer is natural oil. Such oils lock moisture in more efficiently than any petrochemical, and in the meantime accelerate the skin's own repair process. Some of the most beneficial oils for your skin are coconut, jojoba, grapeseed, rice bran, olive, and shea butter. They work to strengthen the skin's own protective barrier, and nourish skin cells with essential fatty acids. Although water is often the most abundant ingredient in a moisturizer, it does not do our skin any good. In fact, high water content in a cream or a lotion is worse to our skin than high oil content. In the next chapter you will learn why plant oil is your skin's best friend and how you can use wonderful oil combinations to heal and protect your skin.

Another goal of modern-day moisturizers is encouraging the skin to generate its own natural moisturizers. Alpha hydroxy acids (AHAs) like glycolic acid and lactic acid help dry skin restore itself in partly by sloughing off dead skin cells, but in high enough concentrations (at least 2 percent) and chemically effective formulas, they actually stimulate the skin's production of hyaluronic acid—a naturally occurring humectant that can hold up to one thousand times its weight in water. But if you have sensitive skin, you should approach acid-containing moisturizers with caution, as they can trigger sensitivities that can be quite intense. Never combine fruit acids with vitamin A derivatives, which you can identify as "retinol" or "retinyl" in the ingredients list.

For the maintenance of the skin's barrier, nothing does as good a job as the skin can do for itself. As you work to protect your skin from moisture loss, you allow it to become healthier and resilient on its own. Here are some tips to making your moisturizing cream or lotion work best for your skin:

1. Never apply the moisturizer on damp skin. Of course, we all have seen those commercials that recommend applying a moisturizer on damp skin "to lock in moisture." This only works if you are applying neat oil. If you apply a moisturizer (which is already made of 50 percent water) to damp skin, you only dilute all those beneficial ingredients, so you end up with a thinner layer of moisturizer after the water has evaporated. To reap all benefits of moisturizer's oils, humectants, and emollients, pat your skin dry after cleansing or toning and only then apply a dime-size amount to your face.

2. Always apply a moisturizer using upward strokes. In two or three weeks you will notice that your skin has become more toned and resilient. Pulling your skin down only helps the gravity to sag your skin even more.

3. Moisturize your environment too. Install a humidifier and fill it with distilled water, possibly adding a few drops of your favorite essential oil. Plants help normalize the humidity levels too. Choose leafy, rich green varieties and definitely not cacti! For a quick and cheap humidifier, place a dish filled with water and possibly some essential oil near or under the radiator.

4. Don't be afraid to mix and match your moisturizers, serums, and night creams, as long as you don't apply acids and vitamin A at the same time. There's nothing wrong in combining a moisturizer from one brand with a serum from another one, as long as they both work well for your skin. To avoid spending lots of money on ready-made facial oil, turn to the next chapter, where you will find amazingly effective recipes for treatment oils for your skin type.

5. Always do a patch test on the inner side of your elbow if you are thinking of buying a new moisturizer. You can encounter an adverse reaction even to a well-known brand or a pure organic balm containing only "skin-friendly" butters. Our bodies are put on high alert due to all the chemicals attacking our immune systems. There's no chance of predicting how your skin reacts to even the most nonthreatening ingredient. Even chamomile, green tea, beeswax, and olive oil can trigger sensitivities in some people. Always try to obtain a sample of a new product to give it a good try before you buy. At least, ask for a permission to decant a small amount to your own clean jar—most stores will be happy to help. Just a reminder: avoid parabens, petrochemicals, alcohol, and artificial fragrances (masking under "perfume" on the label) to ensure your skin's healthy looks for many years ahead.

Of course, the greenest and most cost-effective way to combine all the best ingredients in one moisturizer is to cook one from scratch. Making your own moisturizer at home is difficult, but it can be done. For complete instructions you can turn to my book, *Green Beauty Recipes: Easy Homemade Recipes to Make Your Own Organic and Natural Skincare, Hair Care and Body Care Products*. If you can make custard or béchamel sauce, you can make face cream.

NATURAL SUN PROTECTION

We are all brainwashed to believe that we need sun protection 24/7, even in winter, even when in the underground garage, definitely on our eyelids and lips, and optionally on the nails. But going extreme with sun protection is not going to guarantee you comprehensive insurance against wrinkles and skin cancer.

In fact, frequent use of sunscreen has been shown as a risk factor for the deadliest form of cancer, melanoma. What happens in reality is that people covered in sunscreen tend to stay out in the sun carelessly, for much longer than in the olden days when an extra five minutes under midday sun would mean painful and embarrassing sunburn. Another reason lies in conventional sunscreen formulations themselves. To begin with, most chemical sunscreens, such as benzophenone varieties or cinnamates, are allergens and estrogen mimickers. To work their magic, they need to penetrate the skin, where they start a complex chemical cookery session with the sun's rays, with leftovers poured into our bloodstream. During these chemical reactions with UV rays, our skin becomes more vulnerable to free radicals. Second, most sunscreens are loaded with potentially toxic chemicals including petrochemicals, preservatives, and artificial fragrances, which enter our bloodstream more eagerly in hot humid summer conditions. And third, nearly every chemical sunscreen on the market contains a dangerous form of vitamin A, retinyl palmitate, which may increase skin damage by free radicals and make it more susceptible to dangerous effects of UV radiation.

Do we need to skip sunscreens completely and embrace the sun? Of course not. Sun rays today are not the same as they were fifty or even twenty years ago. The ozone layer was thicker, and there was less pollution in the air. A sun-protecting cream with minimum SPF 15 is absolutely a must if you head anywhere sunny and hot—or if you are off to a ski holiday. The damaging effect of sun rays multiples when we are near reflective surfaces such as water, white sand, or snow. Sun rays are also more active at high altitudes, so you should use at least SPF 30 when you are over six thousand feet above sea level or when your airplane seat is near the window.

But do you really need sun protection in the winter, especially if you live in gloomy climates with little chance of sunshine? The British Association of Dermatologists warned in their 2012 human trial that heavy use of sunscreen severely depletes vitamin D levels.[125]

Sun protection creams made purely with zinc oxide are hard to find, but they exist. If all fails, you can turn your regular moisturizer into a mineral sunscreen quite simply. First, you need to buy some cosmetic-grade zinc oxide—for helpful hints, turn to Appendix B. You will also need a lightweight organic face or body lotion (organic baby lotions are the best). To provide SPF 25 or 30, you need at least 20 percent zinc oxide concentration. Now do your math. For 100 mL (3.3 fl. oz.) of a base cream you need 20 g zinc oxide. That's roughly 4 tablespoons—of course, you can measure more precisely using electronic kitchen scales, but I prefer to go a little overboard when it comes to zinc oxide. Here's what to do next:

1. Measure 100ml (3.3 fl. oz.) of the base lotion into a bowl.
2. Stir in 3–4 tablespoons oil (I prefer extra virgin olive oil) into the zinc oxide powder. Blend well. Zinc oxide will make your lotion a little bit drying, so the oil will compensate for this. This step ensures that zinc oxide dissolves better in the lotion so that the whitish cast on the skin will be less visible.
3. Whisk well to avoid lumps and grits. If the powder does not dissolve too well, add a little more oil— but not water. Wait two to three minutes and then whisk again.
4. The texture should be similar to thick custard, but the cream should glide easily over the skin. If the cream feels heavy, you can add a few drops of oil and whisk well again.

People with darker complexions are not huge fans of natural sunblocks because of the white residue minerals leave on their skin. While lighter skin tones can get away with a light tint of their sunscreen, darker complexions can neutralize this effect in two ways. First, you can add a pinch of a rich, dark mineral bronzer powder to the base cream when you add zinc oxide. Mineral bronzers contain titanium dioxide, which adds to the overall sun protection of your cream. Blend well and test the resulting shade—you may need to add more bronzer if you prefer an iridescent finish. The new tinted sunscreen will be only suitable for use on the face—but of course you can easily make a new non-tinted batch to use on the body. Alternatively, you can apply the sun cream as is and add a swipe of a bronzer or a mineral foundation on top of the cream—again, it will also increase the natural sun protection factor of your homemade sunscreen.

As an emergency solution, you can use diaper rash cream with zinc oxide—for many years, this was my refuge, as I didn't want to use chemical sunscreens yet wanted to use natural sun protection. Zinc oxide in baby creams is usually less than 20 per cent required for SPF 30 protection but it's still better than nothing. More sophisticated zinc oxide protection is offered by such brands as Raw Elements and Badger (there are more suggestions at the end of this book). Some natural and organic sunscreens contain aluminum salts so I recommend you always read the ingredient list for hidden dangers.

Today, to ensure comprehensive sun protection we must "sun-proof" our skin from inside and out. Before your summer vacation, or year-round if you live in a sunny climate, pop a lycopene supplement and eat lots and lots of tomatoes, carrots, and watermelon. Lycopene is a powerful scavenger of free radicals. When it comes to sun protection, lycopene protects against UV damage of skin DNA and may even help ward off long-term photodamage such as uneven color and thicker texture of the skin after too much sun exposure. The richest source of lycopene is tomato paste, which can be used in endless varieties of pasta sauces and risottos, added to soups and casseroles, and even spread on toast with a drizzle of olive oil. In a British study that first demonstrated rejuvenating qualities of tomato paste,[126] participants ate 55 g tomato paste a day, with some olive oil, so why not follow their lead?

SMOOTH AND SHINY LIPS

Did you know that your lip gloss is a great-great-grandson of the first-ever cosmetic product created? Lip decorations with precious stones were used by women in Mesopotamia dating back to 3500 BC, while ancient Egyptians used seaweed and iodine to add color to their lips. Since the mid-1800s, most lipsticks were colored with lead-containing pigments, and this practice continues today despite numerous scientific studies dating back to the 1850s about dangerous effects of lead on human health. Lipsticks, lip glosses, and lip balms are mainstays in any woman's beauty stash, and they are thankfully easy to make at home. All you need is a chunk of a solid butter such as cocoa and a few drops of vegetable oil. You can also add a pinch of any mineral glitter to the melted cocoa butter to create your own custom-blended and absolutely natural lip color. For mineral pigment sources, please check the appendix at the end of this book.

I found that a half-teaspoon of golden-rosy mineral glitter dissolved in 1 tablespoon of cocoa butter keeps my lips bright, smooth, and shiny all year long—and I do not risk swallowing any mineral oil, artificial dyes, phthalates, or lead-containing pigments found in many conventional lip products.

To achieve beautiful lips, you don't need to suffer painless injections or spend untold time reapplying "volume-boosting" lip gloss that almost always has an acrid smell of synthetic mint. Here are simple one-step tips to keep your lips supple and glowing:

1. After cleansing your face, pour a little oil (olive, grapeseed, or jojoba) facial oil onto an old, clean

toothbrush and gently polish your lips. Massage the remaining oil into the lip contour.

2. Castor seed oil is an overnight remedy for cracked, chapping lips. So is organic, unprocessed honey.
3. Rub your lips with the inside of a mango skin—and, of course, feel free to eat the flesh. Mango pulp contains vitamin C and exfoliating enzymes that gently dissolve dead skin cells. You can also try this trick to give your complexion a serious fruity peel.

Persistently dry, chapped lips can be due to dehydration or not enough essential fats in your diet. Breathing cold, dry air through your mouth and licking your lips can leave them sore and chapped, so make sure you always wear a lip balm that is not scented with vanilla or fruity, foody scents. The yummier your lip product, the more prone you are to licking your lips subconsciously. I find that lip balms and glosses with beeswax tend to form a ridge around my lips in cold weather, so if you are as spoiled for choice as I am, then try wax-free vegan lip balms from Aubrey Organics, Merry Hemsters, or Eco Lips.

Cracked lips and dry, peeling cuticles can also be a sign you are low in B vitamins. Take a supplement to get rid of the cracks quickly. Eat beans, peas, lentils, free-range unprocessed meat, and dairy. If your lips are naturally colorful and free from chapping or painful cracking, you probably won't even need lip color.

NATURAL SPA FACIAL AT HOME

Your skin and overall facial contours show signs of stress more quickly than any other part of the body. When we suffer from chronic stress, the downward grimace of low mood and anxiety literally pulls our faces downward, accelerating the formation of nose-to-mouth folds and creases. So having a weekly destressing facial not only improves your skin tone and clarity, it may also diminish the damage the stress and less-than-healthy lifestyle have already done. And if your face feels brighter and younger, your mind will follow the lead!

If you are on a budget, or working to pare down your beauty routine, you don't need to go to a spa for a facial. Using simple kitchen staples such as fruit, vegetables, oils, and salt or sugar, you can replicate spa results without paying a huge premium for luxury packaging—and, needless to say, you won't expose your skin to synthetic chemicals abundant in most spa skincare products. By making your own masks and scrubs you can achieve wonderful results.

Start your weekly facial with a good cleanse to remove makeup and daily grime, and follow with an exfoliating treatment. If you have acne or tender skin, scrubs with abrasive particles can damage your skin even further. Use natural acids like citric, acetic, or lactic, found in lemons, apples, yogurts, and strawberries, to name just a few natural glow boosters. Simply mashing or grating some fruit and spreading the pulp over your skin, then rubbing it off with circular massaging motions, will remove dead skin cells and impurities without damaging the skin. Applesauce, possibly with added fine salt or sugar, makes a super-easy skin exfoliating mask.

After exfoliation, rinse and pat skin dry. If you have ten minutes of time to spare, you can treat yourself to a fragrant facial steam bath. Simply pour some very hot—not boiling!—water over any fresh or dry herbs you have at your disposal such as dill, lavender, chamomile, rosemary, or sage. Feel free to experiment and combine the herbs to your liking; there are no set rules here. Do not think that you will make your steam bath more effective by using boiling water that produces lots and lots of steam. You won't be able to absorb all the goodness in that steam because it will be too hot and may even scald your face; however, simple hot water will produce just enough steam to gently cocoon your face with evaporating essential oils and precious volatile compounds from the herbs so nothing is lost in thin air. Allow the vapors to caress your skin for eight to ten minutes, then gently pat face dry with a washcloth or muslin cloth.

Here's a shortcut if you want to deep-cleanse and treat your skin but have no time (or herbs) for a proper steam bath. Make 2 cups of green tea, and then pour them on a clean towel—a hand towel would do. Make sure it's not too hot. Place the towel on your face and relax for five to ten minutes while thinking positive, calming thoughts.

Now it's time for a mask you can prepare yourself from ingredients that are most suitable for your current skin condition. If you want to purify and deeply cleanse your skin, use white or green clay, which you can buy in bulk and store in a jar at home to use in your homemade beauty products. The rule of thumb is to add one measure of liquid to two measures of clay, but please feel free to experiment, as long as you achieve the consistency of a smooth paste that won't run off your face. Here are some one-step deep-cleansing face mask ideas:

> **Green tea and clay**: Combine 2 tablespoons of green or white clay with 1 tablespoon freshly made green tea.
>
> **Get juicy**: Add citrus, tomato or apple juice to clay to clarify and brighten your complexion.
>
> **Cooling clay**: Peppermint tea and clay make an astringent mask that is excellent for oily skin.
>
> **Witch hazel and clay**: This traditional combination works wonders on acne and blemishes.

If your skin is on the sensitive or dry side, it will benefit from less trying bases for your mask. Think honey, aloe vera gel, live natural yogurt, or fruit purées. You can add more substance to your mask with a little cornstarch, rice flour, vegetable shortening, or dry milk powder. All of these masks can be kept on your face for up to twenty minutes or as long as they feel comfortable. Here are some easy ideas from your kitchen:

> **Nourishing face mask:** Mash 1 banana and combine with 1 teaspoon of honey.
> **Brightening face mask:** Grate 1 raw potato, squeeze the juice and combine with just enough rice flour to make a smooth paste.
> **Green goodness mask:** Combine 2 tablespoons applesauce with ½ teaspoon spirulina powder, and then stir well.
> **Healing skin mask:** Soothe a sunburn with 1 tablespoon aloe vera gel combined with 1 teaspoon honey; if the mask feels too runny, add some cornstarch or rice flour.
> **Berry galore mask:** Raid your fridge and mash together any berries you find. Raspberries, strawberries, and blueberries will lightly exfoliate and brighten your skin while infusing it with glow-boosting vitamin C.

After you have spent at least ten minutes with the mask of your choice, rinse it gently with tepid water, and pat face dry. Look in the mirror and adore the glowing, relaxed, smooth face of a new you!

Chapter Six Quick Tips

1. **Make your own beauty products**—it's a lot easier than you think and will save you quite a lot of money too. Plus, you will know exactly what goes in your lotion, shampoo, or scrub. Flex your cosmetic formulator muscle by experimenting with masks, toners, and simple shampoos based on castile soap, and after you feel confident enough, try making your own creams and cleansers.

2. **Double cleansing is essential for glowing skin.** Combine two cleansers, one to remove daily grime and another one to deeply cleanse and purify your skin. Choose cleansing oils if your skin is dry or sensitive.

3. Cleansing clays are excellent for oily skin: **add clays to your daily cleanser and makeup remover and make a deep-cleansing clay mask once or twice a week.** Choose aluminum-free clays such as fango, montmorillonite, or rhassoul mud.

4. **Use toners**—even if the current cosmetic trend advises you that toners are out of fashion. A plant hydrosol or green tea infusion will not only remove all traces of cleanser from your skin, but will also leave a thin, nongreasy film of beneficial phytochemicals and essential oils.

5. **Scrub and exfoliate with care**: choose nonabrasive, fruit- and lactic-acid-based treatments if your skin is dry, delicate, or inflamed, and feel free to experiment with fine salt, sugar, semolina, or crushed fruit kernels if your skin is oily or combination.

6. **Moisturize and protect from the sun**: these two steps will ensure your skin will glow and radiate health and vitality. Choose mineral sunblocks that

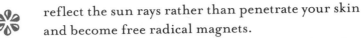

reflect the sun rays rather than penetrate your skin and become free radical magnets.

7. Natural oils and butters are your lips' best friends. Beeswax tends to dry the skin a little. **If your lips are inflamed, cover them with honey and leave it overnight.**

8. **Once a week, treat your skin with a relaxing, deeply conditioning spa facial** complete with exfoliation, steaming, a purifying clay mask, and a moisture-boosting fruit pack.

SEVEN

Beautifully Spotless Skin

Oily skin can happen at any age. For many of us, oily skin and its ugly sister, acne, almost always conjure up thoughts of our teenage years. But as someone who spent ten years fighting acne and the next ten years erasing its ugly residue in the form of scars and discoloration, I am aware that blemishes have nothing to do with your age. Your diet, stress levels, hormone fluctuations, and synthetic skincare can make acne happen when we least expect it.

CLEAN SKIN SOLUTIONS

Common acne triggers include sugar, wheat, and dairy, as well as artificial colorings and preservatives in the processed foods. If you suspect your skin becomes oilier after certain meals, try excluding these food categories from your daily diet for a few days and see how your skin feels and looks. In the meantime, add the following acne-busting supplements and nutrients to your daily meals:

Fiber: Bulk-forming "roughage" keeps your bowels working smoothly, absorbs any toxic junk that passes our lips, and reduces the dangerous accumulation of estrogen hormones in the body. You may notice that acne flares up most often after a bout of constipation. The easiest way to consume more fiber is to start your day with an old-fashioned porridge or a fancier version called "Birchermuesli," which is oat flakes soaked overnight in plain water and topped with lots and lots of berries and nuts.

Nothing beats zinc when it comes to blemish reduction. Zinc works to normalize hormonal levels and also to reduce inflammation. Other skin-clearing supplements to consider include a complex of B vitamins, sulfur, and magnesium.

Essential fatty acids, such as one or two tablespoons of cold-pressed flax seed oil a day, help quench low-grade inflammation in acne-prone skin.

Helpful herbs for oily, acne-prone skin include dandelion (a great liver tonic), echinacea (excellent for general immune support), and burdock root (great for hormonal balance and blood purification).

I won my victory over acne six years ago by accident. I started taking a regular valerian herb supplement to help me cope with a new puppy who was a terrible sleeper. After a week of taking valerian twice daily, I suddenly noticed that my skin was free from blemishes. Oily skin and stress levels are linked more intimately than you think.

CLEAN SKINCARE FOR CLEAN SKIN

If you take just one bit of advice from this chapter, make it this: be extra gentle to your oily skin. Ditch alcohol-laden toners and caustic cleansers. Instead, treat your oily skin as if it is recovering from first-degree burns and use products with potentially irritating vitamins and essential oils only where needed, and very sparingly to treat a spot, not the whole face.

You can easily transform any beauty product you currently own into an acne-specific one using purifying, anti-inflammatory essential oils such as tea tree, rosemary, geranium, and lavender. Green clay (bentonite) is very useful to have around if you are prone to oily skin. You can add it to cleansers, toners, and masks anytime you like.

Wash your skin morning and evening with a very gentle cleanser for sensitive skin or even plain natural liquid soap. Here are some recipes of purifying cleansers for your oily skin that you can easily make at home:

> **Foaming face wash with clay:** Add 2 teaspoons green clay to 100 mL (3.3 fl. oz.) natural liquid soap (castile soap is the best) and shake well. Use as a regular cleanser to absorb impurities from pores, which are generally wider in oilier skin types.
>
> **Yogurt and lemon cleanser:** This is a very gentle clarifying treatment made with 1 tablespoon plain yogurt and a few drops of fresh lemon juice. Combine in the palm of your hand and gently massage into the skin, then rinse face dry.
>
> **Clay and oatmeal cleanser:** Cover 2 tablespoons of fine oatmeal with half a cup boiling water and allow cooling until a slimy, sticky liquid forms at the top of the oatmeal. Collect the goop and add a pinch of clay to make a paste. Massage into your face and either rinse off or leave on as a mask for five or six minutes. Eat the porridge while the mask settles!

After a cleanser, apply a simple toner made with one or two ingredients. Avoid alcohol in your toner at all costs. Instead, use witch hazel, tea tree hydrosol, or lavender distillate to remove

NOT ALL OATMEAL IS CREATED EQUAL

Here are four types of oatmeal you can find in supermarkets and health food stores today.

1. *Instant oatmeal. This is the least beneficial type of cereal. Oat has been flaked and chemically processed so nearly all nutrients are gone. To make it up for the lack of taste and goodness, manufacturers add vitamins, sugar, and salt.*
2. *Quick-cooking oats. Grains are not powderized like instant oatmeal, so there are some vitamins and minerals remaining in the cereal. The result is short cooking time and softer consistency. Nutritionally, it's a slightly better choice, but it's still not real oatmeal. On the good side, quick-cooking oats make lovely soft scrubs and face masks.*
3. *Rolled oats. The oats have been steamed, rolled, and pressed so they will cook more quickly. Much of the nutrients are preserved. Rolled oats are very good for general cooking, baking, and for use in skincare recipes.*
4. *Steel-cut oats (aka Irish oatmeal). This is the traditional and most beneficial variety of oatmeal. The grains are not steamed or hulled; they are simply cut with a super-sharp knife to make them easier to cook. All nutrients and fiber content are preserved. On the negative side, this type of oatmeal takes longest to cook—up to thirty minutes!—and it is not very suitable for the use in skincare recipes.*

any cleanser residue and create a very thin, non-comedogenic layer of purifying phytochemicals on the skin surface. Here are some really easy toner ideas:

Witch hazel and clay toner: This dual-phase toner needs to be shaken before use. The idea is quite simple: Add 2–3 teaspoons of green clay to a small bottle (100 mL / 3.3 fl. oz. or less) of witch hazel and shake well. To apply, saturate a cotton pad and wipe your face.

Double apple toner: Combine ½ cup apple juice, ½ cup mineral water, and 2 tablespoons apple cider vinegar in a glass bottle. Close tightly and shake well. Apply with a cotton pad, avoiding eye area.

Milk of magnesia toner: To quickly soothe your skin and diminish blemishes, apply a thin layer of plain, unscented milk of magnesia, a common stomach-soothing medication. Allow to dry and either rinse off or leave overnight.

Acne-prone skin can be surprisingly sensitive, so avoid grainy scrubs that will irritate spots. Instead, use apple cider vinegar and lemon juice diluted with water, green tea, or aloe vera to gently exfoliate the skin and diminish the size of the pores.

Do not skip the moisturizer—even oily skin needs hydration. After many years of trial and error, I realized that the best moisturizer for oily skin is very thin, "dry" oils such as chia, cucumber, jojoba, or thistle. These oils must be applied very sparingly—just two or three drops for the entire face. Their fine molecular structure makes them disappear in the skin without a greasy trace, and their rich antioxidant content helps soothe and heal the skin more efficiently than any oil-free, chemical-laden creams would. You can add a few drops of tea tree, lavender, or eucalyptus essential oils to your facial oil to increase the antibacterial potential of the base oil.

After applying the "dry" oil, allow your skin to absorb it fully, and then continue with a mineral sun protection formulated with zinc oxide. If you are using makeup, switch to mineral foundations formulated with zinc oxide and mineral pigments. As described earlier, I cannot emphasize enough: avoid silicones, bismuth oxychloride, or artificial dyes in your mineral foundation.

Treat your oily skin to a purifying facial at least once a week. If your skin can tolerate it, you can apply a quick clay mask every other day. But once a week, indulge in a complete spa-like facial treatment:

1. Cleanse and exfoliate your skin using diluted apple cider vinegar or lemon juice in the following proportion: 2 tablespoons of the acidic liquid per half cup of green tea or mineral water. Apply with a cotton pad avoiding eye area, then rinse off and pat skin dry.

2. Steam your face using an infusion of nettle, peppermint, and chamomile in very hot water (be careful not to burn your skin!). You can easily buy herbal teas to prepare your purifying facial steam. After steaming your skin for eight to ten minutes, pat face dry. Do not rinse your skin.

3. Apply a clay-based mask. You can prepare a paste of French green clay or Fuller's Earth clay mixed with mineral water, green or black tea, herbal tea, or even fruit juice such as orange or apple. Take 2 tablespoons of clay and add 2 tablespoons of the liquid soap of your choice. Adjust the amount of the liquid to create a smooth paste. Apply a thick layer all over your face including chin and upper neck area. If you plan to wash your hair afterward, work the mask into the hairline where acne blemishes often form. Relax for ten to twelve minutes or until the mask dries out, and rinse face well with warm water.

4. Apply a healing mask. You can choose from a variety of fruit and vegetables that you may have in your refrigerator:

Spinach mask: If using frozen spinach, thaw 1 spinach cube and combine with a little cornstarch to create a paste. If using fresh spinach, make a puree using a blender. Apply to your cleansed face and leave to set for ten to twelve minutes.

Applesauce mask: Apply applesauce in a thick layer all over your face and leave to work its magic for ten to fifteen minutes, then rinse and pat skin dry.

Strawberry and blueberry mask: Purée 2 medium strawberries and 4–5 blueberries in a food processor and apply to your skin. You can also use frozen berries. Fruit acids and natural antioxidants work to mildly exfoliate, brighten, and heal your skin.

Potato and onion mask: This recipe can be smelly, but it works wonders on severely blemished skin. Grate 1 raw potato and ½ medium onion, then mix the pulp well. Take a piece of clean gauze (you can also buy ready-made cotton masks) and apply to your face, then cover it with the vegetable purée. This mask visibly reduces redness and diminishes post-acne marks and discolorations.

If you have been plagued with oily, acne-prone skin at some point in your life, or are suffering from acne right now, you must have already spent years trying to fight it with benzoyl peroxide, retinoids, harsh cleansers, and alcohol-based toners. All these treatments only diminish acne symptoms without addressing the real cause of oily skin. Stress relief, a clean, additive-free diet, and natural skincare will help rebalance your oily skin and prevent skin sensitivities that are quite common in people who tried to conquer their acne with harsh chemical methods. Sensitive, easily irritated skin is a sign of whole-body imbalance, and like oily skin, it can be brought to balance with natural, holistic methods.

Chapter Seven Quick Tips

1. Common acne triggers include sugar, wheat, and dairy. Make sure you **know your blemish triggers** and correct your diet accordingly.

2. Retinoids and benzoyl peroxide are conventional acne treatments, but they can leave your skin vulnerable to free radical damage and thus prone to premature aging. **Tea tree oil and other natural antibacterial substances help regulate acne bacteria** without unpleasant side effects.

3. **Fiber and zinc are some of the most helpful nutrients in your quest for clear skin.** Fiber helps maintain regular bowel movements, while zinc regulates hormone levels often responsible for acne outbreaks.

4. **Clay and witch hazel are probably the most effective natural treatments for blemishes.** Clay absorbs excess oil from deep inside the pores, while witch hazel works as an astringent.

5. **Apple cider vinegar also acts as an exfoliant with antibacterial action,** so it purifies and clarifies at the same time, when added to your toner.

EIGHT

Beautifully Calm Skin

Like acne, sensitive skin is on the rise. Most of us can name up to ten substances that give us redness, itchiness, or rashes when they occur in a cosmetic product. For some of us, it's a harsh detergent or artificial fragrance; for others, it's certain essential oils. Even something as benign as aloe vera or chamomile can trigger a nasty rash or an array of blemishes that can look like acne. We are all prone to sudden episodes of sensitivity due to irritations, breakouts, itchiness, flakiness, or redness, but for some people sensitive skin is an everyday reality. Here's a bit of good news: with natural nutrition and irritant-free skincare, you can have calm, even-toned, glowing skin, no matter what your skin type is.

HOW TO CLEANSE YOUR SENSITIVE SKIN

Facial cleansers usually mean a whole lot of trouble for sensitive skin. Harsh detergents, emulsifiers, penetration enhancers, synthetic fragrances, and preservatives can be found even in products labeled as "dermatologist tested" and "hypoallergenic." Cleansers for sensitive skin should always be non-perfumed and free from alcohol, colorants, detergents, or unnecessary additives that may sound good and reassuring but just as well may bring even more misery. Ideally, your sensitive skin cleanser should contain ten ingredients or less.

Sensitive skin cleansers should be meek and mild. If you have sensitive skin that is on the drier side, then you can use a cleansing lotion. If your sensitive skin is on the oily side or if you use a lot of makeup, then choose a liquid non-detergent gel that does not produce a lot of foam because foam boosters can be irritating. Do not wash your sensitive skin with antibacterial soaps made with animal tallow or even natural cleansers made with a high amount of alcohol. For a toner, your best bet is magnesium-rich mineral water such as Evian or Volvic, rose water, or witch hazel.

You can make your own natural sensitive skin cleanser using natural ingredients from your kitchen. For example, fine oatmeal blended with water will gently cleanse and exfoliate. Here are a few easy ideas for sensitive skin cleansing:

> **Baby formula:** Pour some powder in the palm of your hand and add a few drops of water to form a paste, and then massage it into the skin.
>
> **Xanthan gum** or **vegetable shortening**: Prepare a gel using a pinch of xanthan gum per 1 cup water or green tea; alternatively, make custard using a vegetable shortening and mineral water or green tea. Use as a regular cleansing lotion—the gel will emulsify any impurities so you can rinse them off.
>
> **Vegetable oil**: Use it as a cleansing oil to emulsify and rinse off any makeup if you suffer from sensitive and dry skin.

If you buy a conventional cleanser for your sensitive skin, make sure to thoroughly test the product before you buy. Take some product from the tester bottle or a tube and apply it to the elbow crease or your neck under your ears where your skin is most sensitive. Leave it on for one day and see if there's any reaction such as redness, rashes, itch, or any other changes in the skin texture. Feel free to experiment with conventional cleansers even if they are not labeled "hypoallergenic." Most often, meek and mild cleansers marketed for sensitive skin are made "fragrance free" with a hefty dose of chemicals that mask the natural scent of ingredients. And with sensitive skin, the fewer ingredients you use, the better.

MOISTURIZE WITH CARE

Choosing a moisturizer that will do your sensitive skin more good than bad is harder these days than ever before. Most often, sensitive skin products are loaded with mineral oil, lanolin, petrochemicals, and pore-clogging plant oils and butters such as peanut, macadamia, and cocoa butter. Such popular antiaging ingredients as alpha hydroxy acids, retinol, and vitamin C can also irritate your skin. Chemical sunscreen ingredients are also common allergy triggers.

Some of the best and safest moisturizers for sensitive skin are natural oils applied under mineral foundation or a sun protection cream. Oils are nature's best moisturizers since they require no preservatives to keep fresh or penetration enhancers to enter the skin—thanks to the oil's affinity with skin sebum, oils penetrate the skin easily and deliver their strengthening and anti-inflammatory properties right where needed. Some of the best oils for sensitive skin include sweet almond, avocado, evening primrose, olive, and jojoba. Skin reactions to peanut oil and beeswax are quite common, since many people have allergies to peanuts or pollen products without even knowing it.

When choosing a moisturizer for your sensitive skin, look for plant-derived squalane, soothing bisabolol, calming calendula, and cooling cucumber in the ingredient list. Safer preservatives include p-anisic, levulinic acids and to some extent vitamin E, and gluconolactone (a sugar molecule that also moisturizes the skin). All essential oils, alcohol, acids, and petrochemicals should be avoided. All your sensitive skin really needs is a lightweight oil and water.

WATER YOUR SKIN

Water is your skin's best soother and moisturizer. That's why, if you have sensitive skin, you should be drinking more than the recommended eight glasses of water. Sometimes your skin is not truly sensitive but dehydrated, with microscopic cracks on its surface that allow irritants to easily penetrate the skin. At the same time, skin sensitivities often signal high toxic load in the body, and to get rid of it, nothing beats pure water. Water not only hydrates and plumps the skin from within; it also carries important nutrients across the body and flushes out toxins.

Not all water is created equal. From a health point of view, water in plastic bottles contains certain amounts of phthalates leaching from PET (polyethylene terephthalate), especially if the bottles were exposed to sun or cold. Instead of paying premium for what is often just bottled tap water, buy a stainless steel flask (make sure it is marked as BPA free or "free from phthalates," which can leach from epoxy resin lining in drinking bottles) and fill it throughout the day with filtered water. From the beauty point of view, the best water is rich in magnesium, which works wonders for your mood and skin clarity. Magnesium-rich waters include Evian, Vichy, and Volvic. Use them for drinking, in your beauty treatments, and as skin tonics.

In periods of low humidity, your skin can feel drier and as a result, more sensitive to irritants. Humidifiers can help, but they must be properly cleaned. To inhibit mold and mineral deposits, the US Environmental Protection Agency recommends filling humidifiers with distilled water, not tap.

STRESS RELIEF FOR SENSITIVE SKIN

Sensitive skin can be a symptom of a stress overload. You can notice that your skin is more prone to redness, dryness, or acne blemishes during turbulent periods in your life. Try the stress-relieving techniques described in Chapter One, including yoga, meditation, and self-massage. You can also try inhaling calming essential oils such as frankincense, chamomile, lavender, melissa, rose, pine, bergamot, sandalwood, petitgrain, ylang ylang, or vetiver. You can also prepare a blend of your own. Buying individual oils can be expensive, but in the long run you will save a lot of money by mixing and matching the oils to your needs. Here is a simple facial massage technique that helps ease tension in your facial muscles and scalp.

1. Find a quiet, calm place where you can lie down and relax. Take five deep breaths to start the re-laxation process. If possible, place a few drops of an essential oil of your choice on a tissue and in-hale deeply. For the facial massage, you should be using pure plant oil without any added essential oils to it to avoid irritation. You can also use this massage technique to apply a gentle mask or a scrub such as warm oatmeal or honey, if your skin tolerates it well.

2. Relieve the negative tension around your temples by massaging your temples with your index fingers in clockwise motions.

3. Relieve the tension in your forehead: using three fingers, massage your forehead in firm circular motion starting at the center and moving toward the temples. Using upward motions, work your fingers upward to the hairline.

4. Relieve the tension around your eyes: gently tap around your eye socket several times focusing at the outer corner of each eye.

5. Use upward, circular motions to gently lift and relax the cheeks. Avoid pulling the skin. Feel the cheekbones and the jawline and make little circles around them. Use upward swipes aiming at the temples.

6. Don't forget your neck: Starting from the clavicles, stroke the neck using tapping motion. Run your fingers along the expanse of the neck, from the sides to the back and upward to the chin, and stop at the bottom of the lower lip. This gentle tapping activates the feel-good points in the skin so that it feels invigorated, yet calm.

CALMING DIET FOR YOUR SKIN

A detoxifying diet is the best remedy for sensitive, allergy-prone skin. Cleansing diets can bring a lot of relief to the liver and the colon, where most skin sensitivities really begin. For the more adventurous, short-term fasts or juice fasts can bring significant relief from skin allergies. Even drinking water with some lemon juice in the morning can help your liver a lot, while taking more fiber and unloading your diet from artificial junk, refined wheat, sugar, and excessive protein can make incredible difference to the health of your colon.

For sensitive skin, immune-boosting vitamin C has an ideal anti-inflammatory effect. The best form of vitamin C supplement is time-released ester-C (L-ascorbic acid), possibly combined with rosehip and citrus extract. A bioflavonoid called quercetin also works to reduce allergy symptoms and low-grade inflammation in sensitive, easily irritated skin. There are many quercetin supplements available. Vitamins of the B group also work to quench inflammation and rebalance the skin. Vitamin A (the daily intake should not exceed 20,000 IU) and zinc (50–100 mg daily) help prevent allergic reactions by normalizing the body's response to allergens and irritants.

To maintain healthy skin cell membranes, gamma-linoleic acid (GLA) from evening primrose, black currant seed, or borage oils is simply indispensable. It has a strong anti-inflammatory action and also helps improve sebum production to alleviate skin dryness. The effective dose of GLA-rich oils is 200–400 mg a day, ideally split in two doses and taken at breakfast and at bedtime.

A balanced diet is the best skin soother. Eat lots of oily fish, green vegetables, and nuts as well as carrots and whole-grain cereals. I encourage you to follow a healthy diet following the tips in Chapter Four for one month to see the amazing difference it makes to your sensitive skin. To take good care of the skin, we must take care of the whole body.

Chapter Eight Quick Tips

1. Sweet almond, avocado, evening primrose, olive, and jojoba **oils make the best cleaners** for sensitive skin.

2. When your skin is prone to allergies and irritants, **choose products with short ingredient lists.** Few ingredients mean few chances for irritation.

3. **Water is the best moisturizer, inside and out.** Choose mineral waters with high magnesium content to soothe your skin and add skin-strengthening minerals to keep skin balanced.

4. **Use a simple facial massage technique** with unscented plant oils to firm and soothe sensitive skin.

5. **A balanced diet will strengthen the skin's defenses** against common allergens and irritants; gamma-linoleic acid and vitamin C help alleviate inflammation.

NINE

Beautifully Ageless Skin

Wouldn't it be lovely if your face could remain as glowing and supple as it was when you were a child? Vibrant, firm, and full of energy, without wrinkles or spots? Unfortunately, science yet has to discover a magic cure that would painlessly, safely, and sustainably reverse the aging process, but we can use many natural ingredients, nutrients, vitamins, and even exercise to help hold back the years.

Most of us consider the natural aging process a depressing, inevitable fact of life over which we have little or no control. The message that getting older equals failure and regression is supported by powerful antiaging industry selling us everything from antiwrinkle creams to miracle age-rewinding pills to plastic surgery. A quick Google search on the words "antiaging products" produces overwhelming list of 10,600,000 results.

The inevitable process of skin aging begins as early as the mid-twenties. The natural regeneration processes occurring at the cellular level begin to slow down. Environmental factors such as sun exposure, pollution, toxic ingredients in skincare, and our daily diet all affect the speed of the skin aging, showing up as wrinkles, sagging, hyperpigmentation, and broken capillaries.

This fatalistic approach overlooks the importance of our lifestyle and well-being determining our biological age.

We all know someone who looks ten or fifteen years younger than their chronological age. This is because their inner calendar shows their biological age of thirty while their passport may reveal they are well past fifty. Yoga teachers, for example, almost always look far younger than their fellows who do not practice a healthy mind-set or clean diets.

In a nutshell, biological age is determined by a complicated combination of factors such as cells and tissue function, physical structure of the body, and cognitive function. The way we age is in our own hands. A lot of symptoms of aging are a result of our lifestyle. Poor diet and hormonal imbalance bring on hair loss, cellulite, and abdominal fat. Relentless tanning and smoking result in early wrinkles, parchment-like skin, and heart disease. Alcohol consumption adds to the risk of heart disease and obesity. Lack of energy, stooped posture, diabetes, poor eyesight, bad memory—all these diseases that people consider as inevitable signs of aging largely stem from negative living and negative thinking.

Lucky for us, it is quite possible to turn your back on this way to self-destruction—all it takes is paying attention to the way you eat, think, and take care of your body.

AGELESS SKINCARE RULES

Skin is the first organ to show visible signs of aging such as wrinkles, hyperpigmentation, also called "age spots," lack of tone, and dryness. For many of us, those first crow's feet and skin folds often signal that it's time to double or even triple your efforts with wrinkle creams, masks, or even cosmetic injections. Instead of acting on the surface level, let's learn about simple age-resisting steps that do not involve any chemicals or needles. Not surprisingly, many of them have already been discussed!

- Stop stressing out your skin. A shortage of sleep— fewer than six hours on an ongoing basis—harms your immune system and can lead to a breakdown of skin's collagen fibers. Find your optimum "sleep zone," the number of hours that makes you feel and look really good. To boost the quality of your sleep, quiet your mind and stay away from intense mental or physical activity four hours before bedtime.
- Smoking is one of the worst skin-stressing habits. It creates free radicals that are linked directly to premature aging. Research shows that secondhand smoke causes almost the same damage. Other skin-stressing habits include habitual worry and over-consumption of alcohol and sugary foods, accompanied by nutritional deficiencies.
- Excessive sun exposure is another skin enemy. While moderate sun exposure, especially in the morning, boosts the production of age-resisting vitamin D, baking in the midday sun pushes cells to work in protection mode. Afterward, they switch to repair. The indoors-outdoors yo-yo cycle pushes the limits of your skin's capacity to adapt. Pull out your best armor and protect it every day, especially if you are on the beach or up in the mountains, where air is richer in ozone. Ozone is especially bad for skin because it oxidizes the DNA of the cells. This means that cells have been weakened, something that contributes to wrinkles and lackluster skin.
- Be gentle to your skin in spring and in autumn,

when it is at its weakest, having been damaged from a summer of sun exposure and a winter of harsh winds and indoor heating. Adapt your skincare routine to the season, and your skin will suffer from less stress as it copes with changes in temperature or humidity.

- Water is crucial for helping to plump up and hydrate cells, plus flush out toxins, 10 percent of which are excreted by your skin. Water is your body's all-natural moisturizer, so drinking eight glasses a day is a good place to start. But listen to your body and adapt your water intake. Someone with a larger body size or who is very active will need more water. Remember that diluted juices, soups, and herbal teas add to the total water intake while tea, coffee, and alcohol drinks deduct from it. Make sure to drink an extra glass of pure water for each cup of coffee, which acts as natural diuretic.

ANTIAGING NUTRITION

You are what you eat—this adage is never truer than when talking about skin aging because what we put in our bodies will inevitably accelerate or slow down the aging process. As we grow older, we rarely grow wiser when it comes to food choices. Starting from age thirty-five, nutritional deficiencies will directly affect our skin, hair, and nails. Rather than spending a small fortune on antiwrinkle creams and serums, why not first resist the aging from within?

Your skin is a barometer for what's going on inside your body. Nutritional deficiencies as well as poor lifestyle factors such as smoking, alcohol consumption, and lack of exercise contribute to poor circulation and abundance of free radicals inside our bodies. These free radicals lower our immunity and damage collagen tissue causing wrinkles and sagging skin.

The best place to start would be to boost your intake of vitamin C, which is the ultimate beauty vitamin. You have already learned about the beauty-boosting powers of vitamin C. To resist aging, you need to up your intake of vitamin C not just as a supplement but also in naturally available form as well as in your skincare.

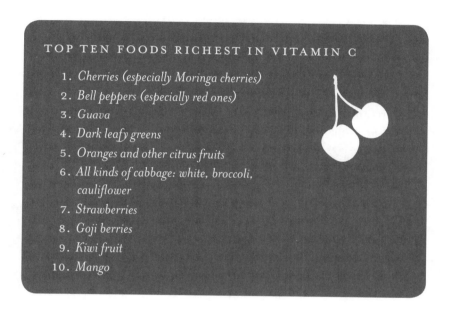

TOP TEN FOODS RICHEST IN VITAMIN C

1. *Cherries (especially Moringa cherries)*
2. *Bell peppers (especially red ones)*
3. *Guava*
4. *Dark leafy greens*
5. *Oranges and other citrus fruits*
6. *All kinds of cabbage: white, broccoli, cauliflower*
7. *Strawberries*
8. *Goji berries*
9. *Kiwi fruit*
10. *Mango*

Often, the nutrients that boost skin health when we eat or drink also deliver amazing skin benefits when they're applied from the outside. Here are the age-reversing foods that also make wonderful addition to your skincare products.

Pomegranate is a true age warrior. Its bittersweet red juice and seeds are bursting with a powerful antioxidant called ellagic acid. Also found in blackberries, raspberries, strawberries, cranberries, walnuts, and pecans, ellagic acid is renowned for protecting and repairing skin cells from environmental damage and UV radiation. Working on a cellular level, ellagic acid keeps your skin glowing by protecting the skin DNA from dangerous carcinogens, including nitrosamines, and polycyclic aromatic hydrocarbons. The easiest way to reap pomegranate goodness is to drink a glass of pure pomegranate juice every day, but for optimum benefits buy whole pomegranates and eat them whole, with seeds and tiny membranes. They contain even more vital compounds for younger skin, including punicalagin to preserve collagen.

Green tea is great for your metabolism and an age-resilient, glowing complexion. All teas contain antioxidants called catechins, along with a host of minerals and vitamins. Catechins have been found to help fight the long-term effects of sun damage, such as sun spots and skin thickening. Ideally, you should drink at least two cups of freshly brewed green tea a day. You can also apply green tea topically as a facial mist or freeze green tea into ice cubes and use them as a toner.

Not many seeds have perfect balance of omega-3 and omega-6 essential fats, which are absolutely essential for keeping skin glowing, plump, and smooth. Hemp seed oil is a rare exception. You can take it as a supplement, or buy cold-pressed hemp seed oil and add it to your salads. Keep in mind that it is not suitable for cooking. You can also put hemp seed oil directly on your skin as a face and body oil. It is absorbed almost instantly without any greasy residue. Thanks to its high levels of polyunsaturated essential fatty acids, hemp seed oil has an anti-inflammatory effect that's an added bonus for those with eczema and psoriasis. The best thing about hemp seed oil is that it helps slow down skin aging. Gamma-linolenic acids (GLAs) in our skin promote regeneration at cellular level, but as we age, our skin loses GLAs and becomes dry and fragile. Hemp seed oil helps replenish these vital lipids. Choose organic, cold-pressed hemp seed oil and try hemp seeds as a protein-boosting snack.

Our skin loves soy milk, even if your taste buds don't! Soy milk is bursting with antioxidants known as isoflavones which work by mimicking estrogen, the hormone used by our body to produce collagen and elastin. Isoflavones also contain in soy yogurts, tofu, as well as lentils, chickpeas, and flaxseeds. You can also use soy milk as a skin cleanser, while soy yogurt makes a lovely, easy mask that improves overall skin elasticity and radiance. Some people notice that regular applications of soy yogurt help reduce skin blotchiness.

Choose good proteins, which are necessary to form collagen, the building block for skin to repair itself. Collagen is also what combats free radicals, those nasty unstable cells that wreak havoc on our skin and ultimately cause wrinkles. Stock your shopping cart with protein sources plus good fats: fish (rich in skin-friendly omega-3 fatty acids), poultry, legumes, beans (also high in fiber to eliminate toxins through the colon), and zinc-packed nuts and seeds. Plus, add foods chock-full of alpha-lipoic acid (brewer's yeast, broccoli, and spinach) to boost skin cells' ability to repair the damage.

Calcium makes our bones stronger but it's also vital to keep our skin wrinkle free (or at least not too wrinkled). Milk and dairy products come to mind first when you think about calcium sources, but there are many other good sources of this vital mineral such as seaweeds, almonds, hazelnuts, sesame seeds, pistachios, beans, quinoa, okra, rutabaga, broccoli, and kale. Figs make an easy skeleton-building snack that instantly provides 250 mg calcium per 100 g dried fruit—that's nearly twice as much as yogurt.

Glowing, smooth skin starts not in a jar of an expensive cream but on a plate and in a cup, so do not delay a visit to the fresh produce counter at your nearest store or, better yet, at a local farmer's market.

DEALING WITH DRY SKIN

Dryness and skin aging are so closely linked, it's impossible to say with confidence which comes first—dehydration or wrinkles. Aging skin is almost always on the dry side, but dry skin can also age prematurely. The dermis layer, which is located beneath the outer epidermis, contains connective tissue along with collagen and elastin fibers that give the skin its elasticity and resilience. Sebaceous glands and blood vessels carry the oxygen and nutrients required to keep the skin soft and supple. As we grow older, the dermis layer becomes thinner and loses its density. As sebaceous glands become less active, our skin is less able to moisturize and protect itself from bacteria and elements. The result is dry, cracked, easily irritated skin.

A classic sign of dry skin is a tight, itchy feeling after you have cleansed, as well as flakiness and pronounced fine wrinkles. Here's how to draw the moisture back in:

1. To cleanse, use non-foaming cream cleanser or a balm that you remove with a cloth. Foam-producing detergents, natural or not, can dry out your skin. You can also saturate your muslin cloth with some oil (olive oil is excellent for this purpose) and wipe off the daily grime, using more cloth and oil as required.

2. Your skin will benefit from a simple toner such as rose water, green tea, or well-diluted pomegranate juice. You can combine all three natural antioxidant fluids for your own highly protective skin mist. After cleansing, mist with a natural face spray,

allow the moisture to absorb or evaporate, and only then apply the moisturizer.

3. Day creams you use should contain sun protection even if you follow them with a layer of mineral foundation. Choose natural sun blocks such as zinc oxide and titanium dioxide and always apply the cream to your neck and décolleté, if needed.

4. Night creams are very useful for constant skin hydration. For best results, your night cream should contain natural antioxidants; vitamins A, C, and E; and hyaluronic acid. To reap maximum benefits, apply your night creams between seven and eleven at night—this is the time when your skin is most responsive to topical nourishment.

It was once believed that the best moisturizer for very dry skin was petrolatum, or petroleum jelly, patented back in 1878. You put petrolatum on the skin, wrapping it in a plastic film so not a single water molecule can escape. These days, petrolatum is used alongside another petrochemical, silicone. All they do is give the skin the attractive sheen and silky touch associated with a healthy complexion, without addressing the real cause of skin dryness.

If your skin feels tight even after moisturizing you need to use little facial oil underneath your moisturizer or a water-free "cold cream"—make sure it does not contain petrolatum, which can make skin dryness more persistent. In the next few pages you will learn how you can easily blend your own "magic potion" to address skin dryness as well other signs of aging.

ANTIAGING POTIONS MADE EASY

Natural, holistic skincare regimen supports younger-looking skin. The following ingredients will help achieve the best results.

Argan oil is the antiaging skincare darling. Unsaturated essential fatty acids in this Mediterranean oil help prevent and reduce inflammation, while moisture-attracting squalane keeps the skin soft. Sterols in argan oil protect the essential protein in the skin, collagen, while antioxidant polyphenols ward off free radicals. Argan oil is safe for sensitive skin and penetrates easily, so you can apply it freely on wrinkles, stretch marks, scars, and discolorations. Argan oil is very beneficial for your skin, so use it generously. If your skin feels greasy, blot the excess with tissue paper.

Avocado oil is rich in skin regenerating oleic acid, vitamins A and D, lecithin, and natural sterols, which help fade sun spots and reduce premature aging caused by excessive sun exposure. To reap maximum benefits, you can apply this lightweight, easily penetrating oil regularly under makeup and in the evening to increase skin hydration and improve elasticity. Avocado oil also preserves the integrity of collagen fibers and helps the skin to remain smooth and glowing.

Grapeseed oil is lightweight, highly emollient oil that sinks right into the skin without any greasy residue. Rich in antioxidant polyphenols from grapes, this oil also helps preserve collagen and resist premature aging resulting from free radical exposure.

Rose hip oil is the champion of antiaging oils. In addition to the high content of anti-inflammatory linoleic and linolenic acids, this oil contains high amounts of vitamin C that easily penetrate the skin, unlike water-soluble ascorbic acid that has trouble reaching lower than upper layers of epidermis. Vitamin C helps strengthen skin capillaries and also maintain strong collagen fibers. To help your skin regain its youthful glow even more quickly, rose hip oil delivers a hefty dose of a natural retinoid, trans-retinoic acid, which combats age spots, scarring, sun damage, and wrinkles. All of these oils can be used straight from the bottle on freshly cleansed skin, or for a relaxing facial massage.

To increase the antiaging potential of these natural wrinkle fighters, you can add one of the following age-resisting concentrates from nature.

Carrot seed oil has a long history of use for wrinkles and loss of firmness. Its rich antioxidant content and presence of natural vitamins A and C helps encourage healthy cell growth, which reduces the scarring and wrinkles. Carrot seed oil gently boosts blood circulation so a healthy glow and improved skin tone appear almost instantly. Carrot seed also helps the skin detoxify itself as it has a gentle depurative (toxin purging) action. To achieve these results, you can add up to ten drops of this sweet-smelling oil to 50 mL (1.7 oz.) of your favorite antiaging base oil.

Geranium essential oil supports a healthy flow of sebum so the skin can moisturize itself. It also has an astringent action, which is great if you have large pores or oily, acne-prone skin. Similar to carrot seed, geranium helps promote blood circulation and protect from free radicals. The unique cellular protection activity of this oil improves skin cell turnover, which tends to slow as we age. Geranium greatly improves the cycle of replacing old cells with healthy new ones. Result? Resilient, smooth, even-toned skin. To reap maximum benefits of geranium, add no more than 10 drops of this oil to 100 mL (3.3 oz.) of your antiaging base oil of choice.

Calendula oil usually comes infused in sunflower or jojoba oil and is an excellent antiwrinkle remedy on its own. Calendula contains high levels of antioxidant flavonoids which protect the collagen fibers from natural decline and even protect the cellular DNA from environmental damage. Calendula oil has a lovely natural bronze tint to it, so you may gently massage it into your skin to achieve a sun-kissed look without harmful sun exposure.

Pomegranate, sea buckthorn, vitamin E, and green tea extracts are also great additions to your antiaging potions, as they help improve skin tone and texture, reduce scarring and discoloration, and even reverse some of the past damage done to the skin.

To reap an almost instant glow-boosting effect, try these easy homemade masks:

> **Lemon tea mask**: Combine 1 teaspoon lemon juice, 1 teaspoon strongly brewed green tea, 1 teaspoon milk powder, and 1 egg white. Beat until smooth and frothy, apply to clean skin using fingertips or a pastry brush, leave to dry, and then rinse.
>
> **Egg and honey facelift**: Whisk 1 egg white and 1 teaspoon honey, apply using pastry brush on clean skin, and leave for ten minutes. Rinse to reveal gorgeously glowing, taut skin.
>
> **Fruity face rejuvenator**: Soak 1 slice of rye bread in little water so it becomes spongy; mash 2–3 strawberries and the bread till smooth, then apply in a thick "crust" all over the face and neck. Leave to dry, then rinse and enjoy a lovely re-energized skin.

GETTING EVEN: DEALING WITH DISCOLORATIONS AND PIGMENTATION

Aging skin is a combination of three factors: sagging skin tone, wrinkles, and pigment patches. Psychologists have found that skin texture and pigmentation affects perceptions of fertility and health.[127] No wonder that, in our quest for glowing skin, we hope to erase all that annoying blotchiness.

Hyperpigmentation, a skin condition characterized by uneven pigmentation, is considered a sign of older age. According to market research by Clinique, one in four of us is concerned with hyperpigmentation, due to increased sun exposure and hormonal imbalances. Many women also experience hyperpigmentation when they become pregnant or start taking birth-control pills.

To determine the cause of your dark spots, take a look in the mirror. Hyperpigmentation in the upper cheek area is often sun induced. This can be easily prevented by regular use of natural sunblock that reflects both UVA and UVB sun rays. Dark patches on your forehead are often a result of hormonal imbalance, as raised hormone levels trigger pigment cells. Spots on your chin and lower cheek area are often a result of acne and careless spot squeezing. In general, oily, easily inflamed skin is also more prone to hyperpigmentation because melanin is distributed unevenly in damaged skin tissue. Skin damage, as minor as exfoliation or upper lip waxing, can also contribute to hyperpigmentation in the lip area and upper cheeks.

Sun exposure remains the main culprit, which is why our hands are the first to show the signs of aging in form of dark spots. To protect the skin affected by patches of pigmentation after exposure to sun, apply natural sunblock with zinc oxide to your hands and neck and use nighttime treatments with licorice and other skin-lightening botanicals described later in this chapter.

Hormone-related hyperpigmentation will fade away naturally as soon as the reason for hormonal imbalance disappears.

Post-inflammatory hyperpigmentation is the hardest to treat. After the skin was damaged, for example, by spot squeezing, scratches, bruises, facial waxing, or chemical peels, clusters of pigment cells travel deeply into the dermis. As a result, darker marks remain after any skin damage has healed. This type of uneven pigmentation requires three-pronged approach: exfoliation to remove dead cells from the skin's surface (this also helps shed excess pigment); mild lightening using safe skin brighteners such as such as licorice and licorice extract, kojic acid, vitamin C, mulberry extract, and niacinamide (they work by interrupting the production of pigment and help evenly distribute melanin cells); and sun protection to prevent new clusters of melanin cells appearing in the treated area. It's especially important to remember that all skin lightening procedures, either by chemical or physical exfoliation or by using melanin-inhibiting botanicals,

remove skin pigment melanin, which has sun-protective properties. Without melanin, skin is even more vulnerable to sun rays.
You can also strengthen your skin's defences by adopting antioxidant-rich diet with lots of lycopene-rich fruit and vegetables
such as tomatoes, carrots, and butternut squash. Lycopene protects
against sun damage and may also help the skin resist premature
aging.

If you are worried not about dark pigment patches but small
veins around the nose and sometimes cheeks, these can be easily
diminished by lifestyle changes. Smoking, alcohol, spicy foods,
and extreme changes in temperature can cause tiny blood vessels
under the skin surface bulge and eventually erupt. To prevent
this from happening, limit your alcohol intake and avoid hot
baths and saunas. Cut back on spices if you think they trigger
skin redness, and eat foods rich in bioflavonoids, such as citrus
fruit and broccoli, which are thought to strengthen capillaries.

Chapter Nine Quick Tips

1. How we live our lives will influence how quickly we
   age. Rest assured that everyone's skin ages, but the
   good news is that **we all have some control over how
   quickly** it does.
2. The high-priced antiaging elixir may sound like a
   good idea (after all, we are "worth" it), but **ageless
   skin is all about how you live your life**.
3. Banish bad habits and **start relaxing and gently exercising** for a glowing skin at any age.
4. Gentle, **natural skincare, regular water intake,
   natural sun protection, and a healthy lifestyle** result in healthier skin texture and firmer face
   contour.

5. **Green tea, calcium, hemp, soy proteins, and**

pomegranate should form the basis of your antiaging skin nutrition, along with ample doses of antioxidants.

6. Carrot seed, rosehip, geranium, and calendula oils are antiaging potions. **Gentle cleansing, and natural toning with plant hydrosols will help keep mature skin in top condition.**

7. **For mild discoloration,** use serums and creams with licorice root extract, which helps to lighten the darkened areas of your skin. **Avoid hydroquinone cream, which bleaches the skin but leaves it vulnerable to UV radiation.**

TEN

Mineral Makeup

Mineral is the only way to go with makeup. It's also the most economical solution. If you take an average drugstore liquid foundation, remove all the silicones, talc, preservatives, triethanolamine, toluene, FD&C dyes, mineral oil, aluminum starch, and artificial fragrances—all those things that damage our health and make our skin prone to aging—you will be left with a pinch of mineral pigments, a dollop of beeswax, and a drop or two of plant extracts.

Meet the mineral foundation. It contains only the basics needed to cover up blemishes and infuse our complexion with a lovely glow. Thanks to the latest technology, minerals can be milled so finely that they stick to the skin's surface without any need for binding and slip agents such as silicones. Since mineral powder contains no water, there's no need to use preservatives either. No wonder mineral foundations, blushers, and highlighters are becoming the makeup of choice for health-conscious models, celebrities, and makeup artists.

Every mineral foundation relies on finely ground stones and sands to help us achieve a perfect complexion. The bulk of a mineral foundation is titanium dioxide, a naturally occurring white mineral that can be found in its purest form in white beach sand. The shimmer comes from mica, while iron oxides add color varieties. Some companies add bells and whistles, such as beneficial plant extracts and zinc oxide for added sun protection, and you already know that zinc has an important role in skin's health, protecting it from inflammation caused by bacteria and oxidative damage.

If there are any health worries regarding mineral foundations, it lies in the texture itself. Smoothness and long-lasting coverage in mineral makeup is achieved by pulverizing or "micronizing" minerals into superfine nanoparticle dust.

Scientists are still trying to come to a definite answer regarding the potential harm of nanoparticles. A large number of studies suggest that insoluble nanoparticles of zinc oxide or titanium dioxide do not penetrate through human skin. A 2012 review of studies on zinc oxide and titanium dioxide nanoparticles said that "cytotoxicity, genotoxicity, photo-genotoxicity, general toxicity and carcinogenicity studies found no difference in the safety profile of micro- or nano-sized materials, all of which were found to be nontoxic."[128]

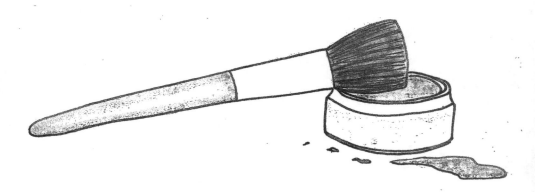

If you prefer to err on the side of caution, stick to pressed mineral powder and fluid mineral foundations that do not require buffing in with a fluffy brush. When you use the powder mineral makeup, please hold your breath while you apply it.

Built-in sun protection is a big advantage of mineral makeup. With an average SPF rating of 15, Bare Minerals has the Skin Cancer Foundation seal of approval as a sunscreen. Jane Iredale claims similar protective effects due to high contents of physical sunscreens titanium dioxide and zinc oxide. But keep in mind that mineral makeup alone will not give you all the sun protection you need. You aren't likely to cover your ears and neck with mineral foundation and even on the face the layer can be too sheer to provide reliable protection. Always prime your skin before applying mineral foundation with moisturizer or sunscreen cream with an SPF of 15 or higher.

Minerals come directly from the earth, so, not surprisingly, mineral pigments are considered some of the most environmentally friendly cosmetic ingredients. Mineral makeup does not rely on petroleum to manufacture its ingredients. Since mineral colors contain no talc, synthetic dyes, preservatives, or fragrance, their carbon blueprint is a lot smaller than that of conventional makeup products. Of course, minerals themselves come from the planet and as any item created by man, mineral makeup involves the use of energy for mining. But unlike iron, coal, diamonds, zinc, titanium, and other ingredients used in cosmetics, they do not require intensive mining such as sub-surface excavation and the heavy use of chemicals. In this way, gram for gram, mineral makeup is a lot less taxing for the environment than conventional foundations and blushers.

You can be green to boot, and reuse sifter jars by buying mineral powders in large "professional size" quantities and decanting them in small, handy pots. For example, you can use a large jar and a large brush for home application of your foundation, and a small jar with a mini "kabuki" brush for touch-ups on the run.

CHOOSING THE RIGHT MINERAL FOUNDATION

Mineral foundations today come in powder and fluid form. Powders are more versatile but less portable. Fluid mineral foundations are less common. Jane Iredale and Miessence make the best ones I have found so far. Fluid mineral foundations are a much better choice for aging skin. In addition to mineral pigments, they contain emollients, humectants, and plant antioxidants, which means that fluid foundations can double as moisturizers. Fluid mineral foundations can be "sealed" with powder mineral foundation, especially if you need to hide birthmarks, post-acne marks, and brown spots. In the summer you can also use Dr. Hauschka Toned Day Cream, which provides quite a substantial layer of natural-looking glowing tint, topped with a mineral powder foundation to strengthen sun protection and prevent powder from accentuating fine lines and wrinkles.

Shopping for the right color is no walk in the park. Here are some tips that you will find useful.

1. **Test the color where you use it.** Always test the color in the middle of your cheek where you can see it. Many sales consultants want you to test the foundation at your neck so that the color "will not leave a visible line." I find this practice useless. People first see your face, not your neck. The foundation must match your facial skin tone. Plus, it's nearly impossible to see your neck clearly in a mirror. For the same reason, don't test for color on your hand unless you are trying to camouflage some scars on your hands.

2. **Step outside.** When you find a color that looks good indoors under fluorescent lights, take a small mirror and walk outside to check the color in natural light. Many mineral foundations appear too shimmery for everyday use.

3. **Add a touch of gold.** Choosing the right foundation color can be tough for women with darker skin tones. That's why most women with dark complexions faithfully stick to their foundations and are reluctant to trade them for mineral versions, no matter how pure they are. Fortunately, most mineral makeup makers have broadened their color spectrum to suit every skin tone. Bare Essentials carries excellent warm and neutral shades ranging from golden caramel to darkest espresso brown. Dark-toned mineral foundations must contain a bit of a golden shimmer to avoid that unattractive ashy effect on dark and olive skin.

4. **Choose the product with the shortest ingredient list.** The more ingredients and products you apply to your skin, the higher the likelihood that mineral foundation may irritate your skin. Choose the simplest mineral foundation formula that does not contain any synthetic additives or preservatives.

5. **Go green.** Mineral foundation should match your natural skin tone as closely as possible, while mineral concealer should be just one shade lighter than your natural skin tone. New mineral powder formulas are specifically formulated to color-correct redness with green undertones.

THE BISMUTH OXYCHLORIDE DILEMMA

Many manufacturers of mineral foundations try to avoid bismuth oxychloride, a once popular mineral salt that produces a subtle shimmer. The Internet is full of blog posts claiming that bismuth oxychloride is terribly dangerous for the skin, and even causes cancer.

Let's set the story straight. Bismuth oxychloride cannot give you cancer.[129] It is not a direct relative of the heavy metal bismuth, and it is not the same as bismuth chloride, which is indeed quite toxic. According to studies published by the Carcinogenic Potency Project at the University of California, tests on animals did not reveal any carcinogenic activity caused by bismuth oxychloride[130]

While bismuth oxychloride has proven antibacterial properties, it can indeed irritate sensitive skin, such as rosacea and eczema patients. Bismuth oxychloride can also aggravate acne, resulting in flare-ups, and even cause the appearance of acne cysts. So, if you are prone to acne or eczema, you may wish to stay away from bismuth oxychloride in your beauty products.

HOW TO BLEND YOUR OWN FOUNDATION

"Bespoke" is a hot word today, just like "green." It is slapped on anything from software to kitchen furniture. Meaning a one-off original, designed and made from scratch, bespoke can also describe made-to-order versions of a manufacturer's standard range.

Bespoke makeup blends are easier to create than you think. You will need to assemble a basic artist's set of paints, or in this case, a few smaller jars of mineral pigments that you can blend and toss together. You will also need a basic paint palette, ideally made of plastic, with round shallow wells, and a few miniature palette knives or spatulas, similar to those found in upscale moisturizers in jars. For precise measurements, invest in a set of miniature measuring stainless steel spoons that can pick exactly a pinch or a dash of fine powder.

For basic blending you will need a small (2 g) jar of each of the following:

- The lightest possible mineral foundation
- Plain golden shimmer
- Plain silver/icy shimmer
- Deep bronze mineral foundation or a bronzer
- Basic rose/pink mineral blush with no shimmer in it

- Optional shades: light green, pale lilac, light pink shimmer

Now you are ready to customize your colors. Clay pigments are best avoided, however, because most mineral clays contain silica and aluminum hydroxide.

Here are some basic combinations that you can use to correct the wrong color, or to tailor the color you've been faithfully wearing for a long time that suddenly feels off. Instead of spending money on a slightly different shade, why not improvise?

If your foundation looks a little bit chalky, it is probably too light for your skin. Maybe you just got a little bit of a tan (and if you read about natural sun protection in Chapter Six, you will know how to do so safely). To correct this, combine a pinch of your usual foundation in a well of the paint palette with a drop of the deep bronze foundation. Add more bronzer until you get the right shade.

If the foundation accentuates fine lines, it's probably too dark for your skin. Combine a pinch of your usual foundation with a drop of the pale one and add two drops of light pink shimmer.

To instantly transform your powder foundation into an oil-free fluid, combine a pinch of your foundation with an equal amount of chamomile hydrosol or witch hazel. Blend carefully in the paint palette.

To instantly transform your powder foundation into a tinted moisturizer with added SPF for summertime, simply blend a pinch of your usual mineral foundation with a dime-size amount of your favorite moisturizer and add two drops of pure golden pigment for added summer luminosity.

If your foundation feels too pink for your skin, add two drops of pure gold pigment and one drop of the palest foundation in your palette and blend carefully. Apply as usual.

If you have olive skin and it suddenly feels washed out, add a drop of pale lilac shimmer and a drop of pure gold shimmer to a pinch of your foundation.

If you are dealing with a sudden bout of redness, correct the problem by mixing a tiny drop of pale green shimmer to a pinch of your foundation. Another solution is to add a drop of pure silver/icy shimmer, but if you don't like too much sparkle, then pale green should work just fine.

To create your own bronzer that will bring a healthy glow without a hint of orange or terracotta, combine two drops of your usual foundation, one drop of pure gold shimmer, one drop of light pink shimmer, and one drop of deep bronze foundation. Blend well and apply sparingly with a blush or all-over fluffy brush. Do not apply bronzer with a kabuki brush, or you will shine like an award statue!

A word of caution: Inhaling mineral makeup particles is not healthy, since titanium dioxide and zinc oxide microparticles can accumulate in lungs. Please avoid fluffing the makeup with a large brush and hold your breath as you blend and apply it.

If you are going to buy just one natural cosmetic product, make it mineral makeup. It is going to sit on your face all day long, so going mineral helps you avoid unnecessary synthetic fillers and preservatives contained in a conventional foundation. It looks more natural too—and we are all for natural perfection, aren't we?

Chapter Ten Quick Tips

1. Choose mineral foundations formulated **without talc, silicones, parabens, artificial dyes, and added fragrances.**

2. For color, **opt for ingredients such as as iron oxides, titanium dioxide, and zinc oxide**, which do not migrate into the skin.

3. Try the color in daylight and right on your face, not on your neck or hand. **Test your colors where you can see them clearly.** If you have darker skin, choose mineral foundations with a dash of gold shimmer in them.

4. **Avoid bismuth oxychloride if you are prone to eczema, acne, or have delicate skin**, as this mineral salt can be quite irritating. Other ingredients to avoid in your mineral foundations include silica (in powdered form), boron nitride, and barium sulfide.

5. **Experiment with mineral foundations** and add them to your daily moisturizer or sunblock to create a shimmery tinted moisturizer.

ELEVEN

Beautiful Eyes

They say that eyes are the windows to the soul, but your eyes can also speak volumes about your general health, your physical and mental well-being. We smile, laugh, and cry with our eyes. No wonder the most important human contact is called eye contact. Maybe that's also the reason why eye creams often cost three times as much as facial creams?

Our eyes cry for more care, and not necessarily in the form of cucumber slices after a heavy night out or yet another slick of eye cream in a desperate attempt to erase those lines. How can we expect our eyes to look bright and beautiful if we deprive them of the uppermost things required for their health: sleep and good humor?

The skin surrounding our eyes is the most fragile on our bodies. Just as the rest of our face, the eye area is constantly withstanding the aging effects of the sun, pollution, smoke, and poor diet, but unlike our facial skin, this skin area has fewer oil glands to remain soft and pliable and fewer blood vessels to remain nourished. That's why you need to double your efforts to nourish your eye area from inside and outside.

1. The eye area is very sensitive, so if there's one product you can afford to buy organic, make it your eye cream. To add extra nourishment to the eye area, set aside a lightweight, "dry" skin oil such as jojoba, chia, cucumber, or argan oil for the use around eyes only. To enrich your eye cream, apply a few drops of the oil of your choice to your fingertips and gently massage (do not pull your skin!) along the eye socket toward your temples. Gentle eye massage also promotes lymph circulation, which helps reduce puffiness and dark circles.

2. Go chic with sunglasses as long as it's not raining cats and dogs. Large sunglasses not only look glamorous, they also protect your sensitive eye area much better. Make sure your sunglasses are protecting from all types of sun rays (UVA and UVB). But most important, choose the ones that look and feel nice. You must love your sunglasses, otherwise you won't be wearing them as often as necessary. Stick to one brand if their frames feel comfortable all day long.

3. Always remove eye makeup *before* cleansing your face. The simplest eye makeup remover is thin oil such as jojoba, sweet almond, or grapeseed, but you can use any oil you have in your kitchen cabinet (as long as it contains no chili peppers!). Saturate a cotton pad with some oil and rub gently aiming toward the temple. Use a fresh pad for each eye—and feel free to use clean sides to remove other long-lasting bits of makeup such as lipstick. Whichever eye makeup remover product you use, take care not to not pull your skin. If you wear

waterproof or long-lasting makeup, repeat the procedure before using your regular face cleansers, which will take care of any makeup remover residue.

EYE LIGHT: DEALING WITH DARK EYE CIRCLES

Dark pigment under your eyes and thin skin that makes blood vessels more visible can be inherited. But it can also be a sign of an iron deficiency, blocked sinuses, hay fever, and plain ol' dehydration. Too much junk food and not enough sleep or fresh air may also be to blame. After questioning my readers, I found that the use of iridescent eye brighteners (think Yves Saint Laurent Touche Eclat or its organic counterpart, UNE Skin Glow Pencil) and brightening eye drops increase on Monday mornings after weekend indulgences in fast food, late nights, and oxygen-lacking air in bars and restaurants. I often notice that sleeping in a bedroom with windows tightly closed will give me not only dark eye circles, but a headache and gloomy mood in the morning—all signs of oxygen deprivation.

Here are some ideas that will chase your dark eye circles to the nearest exit:

1. If you strain your eyes a lot because of work or leisure, make sure to keep your blood sugar levels even. Nothing helps eyes more than regular healthy snacks of whole grain wheat breads and low-glycemic toppings such as tahini, guacamole, or soft low-fat cheese. Cook homemade food at least three times a week. It's not as hard as you think. In most cases, quick-frying a fish fillet and whisking up a quick salad takes fifteen minutes— you'll spend the same time driving to the nearest fast food joint or much more waiting for your meal in a restaurant. And we are not even talking about

saving your hard-earned money by eating natural foods at home! Ensure a steady supply of vital nutrients and you will immediately notice changes in your outlook—literally.

2. Getting out in fresh air will load up your system with oxygen which in turn boosts circulation. Walk at least thirty minutes a day to get your skin glowing. Running makes wonders to your complexion, but if you feel that your skin is flushed after a good run, try another exercise. Broken facial capillaries have never made anyone look better.

3. Blocked sinuses may cause dark circles as well as puffiness. Before you reach for a nasal spray with a solution that will temporarily constrict blood vessels in the area, try sinus-unblocking face massage. Press your skin firmly several times starting at the nose of your bridge, then following to sinus pressure points (located where your nose meets your cheeks) and further toward your cheekbones. To add more interest to the massage, prepare your own sinus-clearing face massage oil by adding 2 drops each of eucalyptus, rosemary, tea tree, and lavender essential oils to 100 mL (3.3 fl. oz.) of lightweight, non-comedogenic oil such as jojoba, grapeseed, or rice bran. You can also try Hopi ear candles to draw out impurities—this reportedly has a good effect on sinuses as well.

UNLOAD THE UNDER-EYE BAGGAGE

Most of us have suffered from eye bags and puffy eyelids at least once. Fluid retention, stress, allergies, hormone changes, and heredity all play their part. One of the most common reasons for puffy eyes is a bout of tears. When we cry, our body reacts to emotions and sends more blood to flow through the eyelids, which leads to swelling. Plus, we pat and rub the area, which doesn't soothe it any more. Paradoxically, too much sleep can sometimes make you look worse. Puffy eyes after a long sleep often result from too much salt and alcohol at dinner, tossing and turning, or a bedroom that is too hot.

Eye puffiness can also result from allergies or irritation caused by eye makeup, eyedrops, and cosmetic products. Try to figure out which product gives you irritation and toss it away no matter how much it cost. An eye cream labeled "hypoallergenic" and "safe for sensitive skin" gave me one of the worst allergic bouts in my life.

Traditional cosmetic offerings for puffy eyes include caffeine-laden creams packed in a roller pen that is supposed to disperse fluids and promote circulation, but this doesn't always do the trick. The caffeine content of such creams is usually too low to make any difference. You will be better off with a cup of espresso—and it costs considerably less.

Green tea de-puffs and firms swollen eyelids. Prepare a cup of green or peppermint tea and let it cool down. Cover the cup with a saucer to prevent precious phytochemicals from evaporating. When nearly cold, pour the tea into ice cube tray and freeze. As needed, wrap the ice cube in gauze or muslin cloth and wipe your eye directing from inner corner outward.

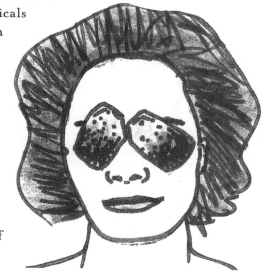

If your puffy eyes are not caused by hay fever, a virus, or an allergy, there are many inexpensive ways to get rid of excess baggage:

1. Wash your face with ice cold water, splashing into eyes to help tighten the skin and promote blood flow. Gently rub your eyes with an herbal ice cube (find the recipe in Chapter Six). If the ice is stinging your skin, wrap it in muslin cloth or a paper towel.

2. The traditional advice is to place two slices of cool cucumber on the eyes for several minutes, but this rarely helps if you are not pressing cucumber slices into your eye sockets. I found that soaking two black or green tea bags in cold water, chilling them in the refrigerator, and placing them over closed eyelids for several minutes works much better.

3. Steaming your face helps purge excess water and tighten the skin. To relieve water retention, add fennel, dill, parsley, or rosemary to the bowl of hot water, then carefully lean over and cover your head with a towel. Steam your face for five to ten minutes.

4. Add celery and parsley to your salads. Herbs that ease puffiness and water retention include dandelion, corn silk, nettle, cleavers, and meadowsweet.

5. Bloodshot, swollen eyes can be due to a lack of vitamin B2. Good sources of this vitamin include eggs, cottage cheese, yogurt, broccoli, asparagus, spinach, mushrooms, brewer's yeast, and almonds.

6. To camouflage puffy eyes, do not pile on shimmery eye shadows. Instead, apply some matte face powder to the eyelid and focus your attention on eyelashes: curl and color them to visually open the eye and distract attention from the puffiness.

FEED YOUR EYES

As your skin needs nutrients to remain resilient and bright, so do your eyes. There is solid scientific evidence that you can protect your vision from age-related degradation by enriching your diet with lots and lots of eye-specific antioxidants, vitamins, and minerals. The best way to obtain antioxidants is from fresh fruit and vegetables—the more colorful, the better.

- Eye-nourishing antioxidants are abundant in purple fruit and vegetables—for example, eggplant, red cabbage, dark grapes, blackberries, and blueberries. They contain flavonoids lutein and zeaxanthin, two antioxidants are responsible for sharp vision.
- Zinc, copper, and vitamin C help protect your vision from age-related changes such as glaucoma. Luckily, these supplements are also known to protect your skin from premature aging and to generally improve your immunity.
- Ginkgo biloba is a well-known herb that helps improve blood circulation and memory. Studies show that ginkgo biloba protects eyesight by maintaining oxygen supply to the eyes and also works as an antioxidant[131]
- Essential omega-3 fatty acids are some of the most important supplements for your skin and eyes. The retina has a high concentration of omega-3, particularly DHA. Omega-3s protect eye cells from inflammation, free radicals, neurotoxins, and environmental aggressors. All good reasons to eat more fish or invest in a high-quality omega-3 supplement.

Chapter Eleven Quick Tips

1. Buy organic eye creams. The skin around your eyes is very fragile and sensitive to synthetic irritants, so **going organic with your eye products should be a priority.**

2. Sunglasses are the first warriors of aging skin around the eyes. No matter what the current fashion, **opt for oversized sunglasses that are marked as providing comprehensive sun protection.**

3. Oil makeup removers work a lot better than gels or creams because they dissolve waterproof and mineral makeup more efficiently. **To remove eye makeup easily, saturate a cotton pad with olive oil and gently press onto your eye, then slide to remove traces of mascara and liner.**

4. Green tea and cucumber are excellent for puffy eyes; **slices of raw potato help lighten under-eye circles** much more efficiently than any eye cream.

5. Zinc, copper, and vitamin C ensure good blood circulation in the eye area and slow down collagen loss in fragile skin. **Drinking enough water helps prevent eye puffiness and droopy eyelids** that result from the eye "yo-yo": puffy lids in the morning, dull and tired in the evening.

6. **Purple-colored vegetables help maintain sharp eyesight and also replenish the skin with antioxidants—** essential for wrinkle prevention.

TWELVE

Beautiful Body

Y ou know how important it is to shower regularly, and I bet you already know or have previously guessed that harsh soaps and heavily perfumed shower gels wreak havoc on your skin by stripping away its natural oils and infusing your body with less-than-healthy substances from artificial fragrances and penetration enhancers. To stimulate your senses and wake up your mind without damaging your health, opt for shower gels made with plant-based detergents and scented with essential oils. Gentle cleansing and a pleasant scent are all you really need from your shower gel. The rest of antiaging, brightening, energizing, and skin-lifting bells and whistles are washed off too quickly to make any difference.

If you are getting used to saving water in the shower for budget or environmental reasons, keep shower gel usage to a minimum too. A quarter-size blob of gel is all you need to clean yourself from head to toe in three minutes or less. Unfortunately, hot water dries out the skin and causes small blood vessels to burst.

If you really crave your hot shower to relax aching muscles and banish the blues, turn down the heat and take a warm bath, but make sure to keep the splashing to fifteen minutes. Anything on top of that will dry out your skin.

SKIN MOISTURIZING MADE EASY

Drugstore shelves sag under the weight of a seemingly endless array of body lotions, but you can moisturize your skin easily and inexpensively at home using just one ingredient.

Any season is good for body oils. Winter calls for the richer texture of emollient olive, grapeseed, and sunflower oils, while summer is the season for dry oils such as jojoba, chia, and sweet almond. They smooth your skin and boost your tan, creating a luminous, sexy glow.

The best time to moisturize is after a shower. Once you have gently patted yourself dry with a towel, you have about three minutes to coat your body with oil or lotion. Apply your moisturizer in generous strokes aiming upward, from bottom to top. Quick application allows your skin to retain the water it absorbed during your shower, increasing the benefits of your moisturizer.

If you must have a moisturizer, weed out natural brands that do not practice "greenwashing"—that is, covering lots of synthetics under an "organic" name—then you will enjoy lovely body moisturizers from Dr. Bronner, Lavera, Weleda, Primavera, Pangea Organics, and my own brand, Petite Marie Organics.

Body oils are the best moisturizers, as they give the most water-locking and skin-nourishing effect per drop, and there's no need for the water, emulsifiers, or preservatives that often make up to 80 percent of a regular body lotion. You only need a teaspoon of oil to invoke a gorgeous glow in your chest and legs, and you can try endless variations of essential oils and mineral body shimmers added to your base oils for a truly fantastic glow.

Soya, sweet almond, extra virgin olive, grapeseed, and peach kernel oils are great all-rounders as they leave a lovely sheen on the skin without sticky residue. Jojoba, thistle, and chia oils are more suitable for oilier skins, which can be overloaded with heavier oils. Such oils are called "dry" as they penetrate instantly without any sheen or residue. For extra-nourishing body buttering, you can try coconut oil: it is solid and is sold in jars, but it instantly melts when it touches the skin.

Here are very simple combinations of essential oils if you want to enhance your body oil with beauty "superpowers":

> **Balancing Blend:** Add 8 drops lavender, 4 drops orange, and 1 drop eucalyptus essential oils to 120 mL (4 oz.) base oil of your choice.
>
> **Purifying Blend:** To control body acne and ingrown hairs, add 5 drops tea tree, 5 drops geranium, and 3 drops lemon essential oils to 120 mL (4 oz.) lightweight "dry" base oil such as jojoba or thistle. For sources, get some useful ideas in Appendix C.
>
> **Antiaging Blend:** Add 10 drops sandalwood, 4 drops rose otto (optional), 4 drops rosewood, and 5 drops grapefruit essential oils to a nourishing base oil.
>
> **Aphrodisiac Blend:** Combine 10 drops grapefruit, 8 drops ylang-ylang, 3 drops patchouli, 2 drops vetiver (optional), and 4 drops rose otto in 120 mL (4 oz.) lightweight base oil.

If you come up with a combination of scents that's particularly appealing to you, make a careful note of ingredients that you have used. To prevent your oil from going rancid, store in a dark glass bottle and add 3–5 capsules of vitamin E oil or 2–3 capsules of evening primrose (starflower oil) to your oil. These supplements are available in many pharmacies and health food stores. To use, carefully puncture the capsule with a needle or manicure scissors and squeeze the contents into the container with your oil.

To keep your skin supple and glowing, up the moisture level of the air around you. Dry air sucks the moisture from the skin so it feels dry and taut more quickly. These days, you can find air humidifiers at all price levels and with many useful features such as ionic air-purifying functions that kill airborne bacteria. But the simplest and probably most effective air humidifier is a bowl of water placed near a source of heat. To make the bowl of water more interesting, why not add a floating tea light or a few drops of essential oils?

BODY EXFOLIATION

To help your skin absorb your moisturizer or body oil more efficiently, regular exfoliation is a must. Leave the loosely grained, pleasantly scented scrubs to your face. Body brushing is all your skin needs. When performed daily, it helps purge all those toxins accumulating in fatty tissue, stimulates the circulation, and maintains healthy collagen production. By removing dead skin cells body, brushing makes it easier for the skin to absorb moisturizers and treatment products.

The secret to good body brushing is the right tool. Avoid brushes that scratch your skin: mini tears on your skin surface can lead to maxi inflammation. But remember that too soft won't work either.

One of the most affordable and versatile tools is a loofah. A loofah is made of dried plant fibers and is most effective when wet. It is used strictly to dislodge the dead skin cells that clog pores and give the skin a dry, flaky appearance. Work in circular movements, from your feet to your neck, to help stimulate your circulation. After using it, simply rinse it in warm water and suspend it above a heat source to dry. Replace your loofah regularly as it will lose half of its exfoliating power after three or four months of use.

An exfoliating mitt is used dry to soften the skin and unblock oily pores by stimulating blood flow. Unlike the loofah, the mitt must be treated with care: after use, wet only its surface with a stream of boiling water and then lay it flat to dry. Mitts can grow mold if soaked through.

You should brush before you shower or take a bath, preferably every morning, to boost your mind and spirit. Start at your feet and brush using long, smooth movements working up your legs and across your thighs, hips, and bottom. Move up your arms to the shoulders. Don't be too enthusiastic with the brush, especially if your skin is delicate or you have lots of broken capillaries. Never brush your tummy or bust area. Brush for at least two minutes, then rinse the brush and enter the shower or the bath.

If body brushing is too vigorous a procedure, you can make your own body scrubs. They come in two forms: with exfoliating granules that slough off dead skin cells, or mild acids such as glycolic acid, fruit acids like AHA and BHA, or salicylic acid to dissolve dead cells. Exfoliating once a week will boost your skin's natural regeneration process, smooth and soften your skin, and give you a more radiant complexion. Making your own body scrubs is incredibly easy. If you can make salad dressing, you can make a lovely body scrub too. Here are some ideas to get you started:

> **Coconut Sugar Scrub:** Combine ½ cup fine or raw sugar, ½ cup grated coconut, ½ cup olive oil.
> **Fruity Body Peel:** Mash 1 mango and add juice of ½ lemon; stir well. Use as a scrub if you cannot tolerate grainy exfoliating products.
> **Yogurt Body Exfoliant:** Combine 2 cups plain yogurt with ½ cup oatmeal or semolina flour and 2 tablespoons honey. Stir well and apply generously. This recipe is suitable for sensitive skin.
> **Smoothing Salt Scrub:** Combine ½ cup salt, ½ cup kaolin clay, and ½ aloe vera gel. You can leave this scrub as a body wrap for five to ten minutes if you suffer from cellulite—and who doesn't?

NATURAL TIPS FOR CELLULITE

Stress, poor digestion, and lack of sleep can cause the ripening of "orange peel" and "wobbly bits," as Bridget Jones famously called one of our top body worries. You can also blame it on hormones or synthetic hormone mimickers. Cellulite is affecting us at higher rates and at younger ages than before. Cellulite, a layer of subcutaneous fat, is the culprit behind that orange-peel texture we can get on our stomachs, butts, and thighs, striking skinny and curvy bodies alike. I was stunned to see *very* visible cellulite covering toned hips of a fifteen-year-old pro tennis player. Hormonal imbalances can play part a too, but the main reason why so many women today suffer from unsightly blobs and bumps at very awkward places may be the abundance of hormone-mimicking chemicals in our environment. Estrogen-like food additives, fragrances, preservatives, and dyes trigger the formation of body fat in the waist and lower body areas. Also, excess estrogen is linked to water retention, which could explain why drinking more water results in expelling more water and, as a result, less visible cellulite.

That's the key: less visible. The female body is programmed to store more fat than the male body, and it's impossible to naturally erase all traces of fat from our curves. No one has yet found a way to banish cellulite for good, but there are a few tricks to minimize its appearance. Not a single cellulite cream, as expensive as they can be, can guarantee you dimple-free skin. Most often, their formulas contain ingredients that cause the skin to swell slightly, making those "dips" less visible. The most abundant active ingredient will be caffeine, since the diuretic action commands fat cells to eliminate water. But these water storages will be refilled easily after you drink some water or eat some soup. Water loss during certain "fad diets" brings fast results, but they are never long lasting.

Regular exercise and a healthy diet are still the best way to get your blood pumping and minimize the look of cellulite. But you will need up to six weeks to see results. You can speed up the process of smoothing those unsightly bumps by detoxing your body from the inside out—and from outside in.

First off, increase your fluid intake. While it seems that the more we drink, the more water ends up in fatty cells, this is not true. By drinking more water, we expel more water along with all those toxins accumulating in our bodies. Green tea is still the best beverage in your quest for smooth, glowing skin. Theobromine in green tea helps the body shed extra fat, which means less "orange peel" look and less sun damage too.

Follow up that cup of green tea with a good, thorough body brushing. Good blood circulation is cellulite's worst enemy, and by boosting blood flow through body brushing, you not only help detox your skin, you will feel a lot better overall.

Experiment with clay and seaweed wraps. You can buy seaweed jelly and kaolin clay in bulk in most health food stores or online (check Appendix C for shopping ideas). To make a clay body wrap mask, add 1 measure of green tea, water, or even fruit juice to 2 measures of clay. Your aim is to achieve a custard-like consistency that is not too runny and not too stiff. Brush your body, towel-dry your skin if necessary, and then apply the clay "custard" or seaweed jelly on the troubled areas. Cover them with plastic film (look for the vinyl-free variety) and lie down under a comfortable throw to keep yourself warm. Drink a lot of water as you steam under the throw because clays and seaweed purge excess water from your skin tissue. After ten to fifteen minutes, rinse off the mask, pat dry, and enjoy glowing, even-toned skin.

To seal the deal, you can now apply anticellulite oil. From my experience, oils work better than gels or creams because they penetrate the skin easier. You can make your own anticellulite blend by adding 10 drops of any citrus essential oil to 100 mL (3.3 oz.) of base oil such as jojoba or olive. Here's a recipe for birch anticellulite oil inspired by a similar product made by Weleda.

BIRCH CELLULITE OIL

Birch has a diuretic and toning effect. Birch leaves have traditionally been used as a tea to cleanse the body of excess water. When applied topically, birch causes fatty cells to purge water deposits making cellulite less visible.

Ingredients
120 mL (4 fl. oz.) olive, jojoba, or grapeseed oil
15 drops juniper essential oil
5 drops rosemary essential oil
5 drops orange or lemon essential oil
A handful of fresh birch leaves

Method
Bash the birch leaves in a pestle and mortar, place in the bottom of a wide-neck bottle and pour the olive/jojoba/grapeseed oil on top of them. Add the other oils. Leave the mixture in a bottle for a week in a cool dark place. After a week, strain out the birch leaves, if desired, or leave then inside to infuse the oil even more.

Use
Massage the oil using firm, circular movements aiming upward into the problem areas such as tummy, thighs, or upper arms.

Honey massage is extremely effective not just to minimize the look of cellulite, but also to firm and lift sagging skin on other body areas. Honey naturally absorbs toxins from the skin and infuses it with vitamins and biologically active nutrients. You can use pure honey or mix it with a few drops of cellulite-busting essential oils such as juniper, grapefruit, or orange. Warm up 3 teaspoons of honey with 1 tablespoon of olive oil and massage your problem areas using firm upward strokes. You can also leave the honey on the skin for ten to fifteen minutes under a plastic film wrap. Your skin will be glowing and your cellulite a lot less visible.

Now that you've sent your fat cells a clear signal to get packing, it's time to add specific cellulite-busting, fat-purging, collagen-preserving foods to your grocery list. Non-sugary fruit and non-starchy vegetables are best, but some vegetables should be your prime focus. Cellulite-busting foods include broccoli, rich in fiber and collagen-preserving alpha-lipoic acid; asparagus to fill up with fiber and banish bloating; and oranges (what a coincidence!) that beat "orange peel" with antioxidant bioflavonoids, which improve blood circulation. Whole grain pasta and breads also help remove cellulite-causing toxins from the body. Spice things up with cayenne pepper, which improves fat metabolism; turmeric to improve circulation; and garlic to lower blood cholesterol. To finish your cellulite-busting meal, dessert on lycopene-rich watermelon and apricot, potassium-loaded bananas, and antioxidant-rich various berries, which are indispensable in your quest for smooth, glowing skin, head to toe.

THE HOLISTIC WAY TO A SUNLESS TAN

Getting enough vitamin D from sunlight is important, but you don't have to bake yourself under midday sun rays to get more than plenty of this all-important, cancer-fighting vitamin. Experts agree that just twenty minutes without sunscreen in the morning sun will generate enough vitamin D in your body to improve your immunity and strengthen your bones. So if you say you are tanning to fill up on vitamin D, you are just fooling yourself.

There are countless types of self-tanners available today, and they are way ahead of the original smelly, acrid concoctions that produced awkward shades of orange with visible tan lines between your fingers. These days, self-tanners go on smooth, smell great, and produce believable shades of natural-looking bronze. But to make them work, you have to apply so much effort: epilate and exfoliate first, don't perspire, don't shave for a week, don't get dressed for one hour after application (and who has the patience for that?), don't swim, don't bend, don't curse (or you will perspire even more), don't shower, and don't forget to pat your elbows with a clean tissue, otherwise they will be dark. For two or three days of bronze tint that will wash away and leave your skin looking like giraffe's neck, it's just too many don'ts.

Another problem is that finding a decent self-tanner without parabens, artificial fragrances, petrochemicals, and other potentially unsafe ingredients is nearly impossible. Lavera's all-natural, fast-absorbing self-tanning sprays and lotions are a rare exception, while the rest of the self-tanning crowd is loaded with nasties.

The main active ingredient in self-tanners, dihydroxyacetone (DHA), poses yet another problem. Recent studies found that DHA acts as a free radical magnet, attracting unstable oxygen molecules to the skin where they wreak havoc, speed up premature aging, and even put you in a higher risk group for skin cancer. Synthetic or derived from corn, DHA is a menace. Newer formulas of self-tanners work around DHA and use either lower amounts of this tricky ingredient or use other tanning agents such as caramel (which only gives a nice tint that will rinse off during the next shower or onto your bed linen) or erythrulose, the latest generation bronzer obtained from corn, for natural-looking and lasting results. Scent-wise, peppermint and citrus scents are best as long as they are derived from natural essential oils, not lab-created imitations.

For greener souls like me, the best self-tanner comes in a pill, not a bottle. In France, pharmacies carry tons of various "auto-bronzants"—supplements that claim to produce a sun-free tan. Packaged in cute cream jars, these pills are mostly blends of antioxidant carotenoids such as lycopene to withstand sun damage and triple doses of beta-carotene to induce a lovely bronze glow without a hint of orange thanks to the clever blending of various carotenoids. These tanning pills also work to protect our skin from harmful effects of the sun. Lycopene, which is naturally found in tomatoes and carrots, has been linked to improved protection against sun damage.

For visible results, you must take "autobronzant" carotene supplements for at least three weeks. I have tried nearly every variety available, as I am not a huge fan of self-tanners, and I found these supplements to be quite effective. I noticed that very soon my skin turned a pleasant shade of bronze even in the areas that do not normally tan, and I enjoyed knowing that for the first time in my life I am tanning my skin while actually improving my health. Only a few weeks ago, in the middle of winter, I needed to urgently finish a jar of "autobronzant" before it expired. I turned a lovely shade of believable bronze and even had to change my makeup colors to summer palettes. Not many of my friends believed that I stayed away from a tanning salon! But the "feel-good factor" of seeing yourself tanned and knowing that it's harmless is even more precious.

> **Tanning Bath Recipe**: to maintain your tan, take a weekly bath with very strong black tea. Boil 2 cups of dry black tea leaves (any variety will do) in a pan for five minutes, strain, and pour the liquid into the bathwater. (Interestingly, black tea worked as a tights substitute during World War II when women painted their legs with strong solution of black tea.)

BATHE YOUR WAY TO GLOWING SKIN

Thalassotherapy and hydrotherapy are two of the earliest detoxing techniques. Thalassotherapy, from the Greek word *thalass* meaning "sea," is a form of holistic body treatment using seawater and seaweed. During a thalassotherapy session, trace elements of magnesium, potassium, calcium, sodium, and iodide suspended in seawater are absorbed through the skin. Adding seaweed to the seawater can firm the skin and reduce fatty accumulations.

Creating your own seawater spa treatment at home is wonderfully easy. All you need is a packet of Epsom or untreated sea salt (the coarser, the better). Place a few cups of salt at the bottom of the bath and add warm water. Make sure all the salt has dissolved, otherwise your bottom will be treated to some exfoliating salt grits. By adding a cup of baking soda to the bathwater, you will make it softer and more soothing for your skin.

You can easily prepare a seaweed bath at a fraction of the cost in the comfort of your own bathroom. You can collect fresh seaweed during a summer vacation if you are not lucky enough to live near the sea. Dried seaweed is also available in health food stores.

Start your seawater treatment by making the bath environment peaceful and quiet. Light a few candles and prepare a towel and a bath robe. Turn on some tranquil music. The smell of seaweed can be quite strong, so you can add a few drops of lavender or chamomile essential oil. Soak for at least fifteen to twenty minutes, allowing the healing water to penetrate your pores. You will rise to a firmer, glowing skin thanks to the high mineral content of the water. As the seaweed can leave a slippery residue, you may wish to shower after the bath. Make sure to use a rich body moisturizer as sea water treatments can be quite taxing for dry skin types.

Here are some other bath recipes to try:

Green Tea Bath: Add 5–6 green tea sachets in bath water and leave to infuse for five to eight minutes. Green tea will soothe and purify your skin while black tea will invigorate and stimulate your body and mind.

Oatmeal Soak: Pack some oatmeal into a nylon stocking or some muslin cloth, tie the end, and place under running water while filling up your bath. You can also use soft oatmeal to scrub your face and body. This bath is very soothing for sensitive skin types.

Milk & Honey Body Soak: To recreate a famous Cleopatra's milk bath at home, add 5–6 cups of milk powder to the running water. Use buttermilk if your skin is on the dry side. For added benefit, swoosh 3–5 teaspoons honey under the running warm water.

Fruity Bath: Pour a few cups of any leftover juices that may be past their prime in your refrigerator. Diluted juices will energize and lightly exfoliate your skin creating a gorgeous glow.

MAGIC IN A BOTTLE:
NATURAL PERFUMES AND DEODORANTS

What makes us crave a certain scent and reject another? Our personal reaction to a fragrance is based on myriads of factors, from our deepest memories to the current state of our endocrine system and even the day of our monthly cycle. Scents invigorate, stimulate, soothe, and sometimes irritate. Too often conventional fragrances contain too many irritating and even toxic substances, including denatured alcohol, solvents, and plasticizers such as phthalates. The fragrance formula can contain hundreds of volatile compounds, which can trigger dermatitis, headaches, and even asthma. Luckily, these days we can choose from dozens of all-natural perfume brands that craft their scented creations in the old-fashioned way from essential oils, fresh plants and plant distillates, waxes, roots, barks, and grain alcohol. Some of the better all-natural fragrance brands include luxurious scents from Creed, Patyka, Frederic Malle, Il Profvmo, Honore De Pres, and more affordable but still very natural ones from Lavere and

Weleda. For a complete listing of natural fragrance brands, please refer to Appendix B at the end of this book.

Choosing a perfectly natural yet effective deodorant is more difficult. For something used so frequently, don't you want a product that does the job without possibly compromising your health? Conventional deodorants usually contain harsh chemical antiperspirants, which may cause irritation or allergic reaction to the ultra-absorbent underarm skin.

The skin is your body's largest organ and, just like kidneys, is constantly working to rid the body of toxins. Natural deodorants, unlike their conventional counterparts, do not contain aluminum chlorohydrate, which may be irritating to the skin or pose even more serious danger. The fact is, they often work by clogging pores to inhibit a natural function of your body—perspiring—which enables your body to naturally rid itself of toxins that may adversely affect your health. As discussed earlier, nearly all antiperspirants contain various aluminum salts, which are linked to breast cancer and Alzheimer's disease. Even natural deodorants marked as "aluminum free" may still contain a natural aluminum salt called alum (aluminum silicate). If you do not wish to expose yourself to this toxic metal, you can still smell fresh with these simple and natural alternatives.

Bacteria are the source of body odor, and natural deodorants are effective at reducing those bacterial culprits. Some of the ingredients to look for are baking soda, zinc ricinoleate, lichen, fruit extracts, and essential oils from herbs such as sage, tea tree, lavender, chamomile, aloe, lemon verbena, coriander, and lemongrass. Many so-called "natural" deodorants are anything but natural, being made almost entirely of propylene glycol with a few drops of essentials oil.

- Place 3–4 fresh or dried peppermint, bay, or sage leaves (or 2–3 twigs of lavender or rosemary, depending on your personal preferences) in a bottle containing 1 cup water and 1 cup grain or grape alcohol, preferably organic. Allow to infuse for two or three days, and then spray the homemade deodorant under arms after shower. Do not use on freshly shaved skin.

- Combine 100 mL (3.3 fl. oz.) witch hazel and 1 tablespoon apple cider vinegar for a naturally refreshing and odor-resisting blend that you can use anytime.
- Add 1 teaspoon white clay (kaolin) to 100 mL (3.3 fl. oz.) water and 30 mL (1 fl. oz.) grain alcohol. Pour into a spray bottle and shake well before use. Kaolin will absorb scents without penetrating the skin.
- Dust your underarms or other areas that tend to sweat a lot with baking soda, which makes a very effective and nearly invisible alternative to talcum body powders.
- Dust your underarms or other areas with a blend of cornstarch and white kaolin clay.

Just remember, as with conventional products, some people need more protection than others and should plan to reapply deodorant during the day.

You may find that you sweat more after eating certain foods. Deep-fried, spicy, and salty foods such as curry, sweet-and-sour sauces, and dishes with wasabi, as well as chili, jalapeño, and pimento peppers, won't give you a chance to stay dry through the meal. Coffee, garlic, onions, and added salt are major sweat triggers in your diet. Eat well, and stay dry without toxic chemicals.

BLOOMING GORGEOUS:
NATURAL BEAUTY DURING PREGNANCY

Pregnancy is probably the most important period in a woman's life, and staying gorgeous in a natural, nontoxic way is not a luxury; it's a top priority. Unfortunately, many skincare products aimed at pregnant women are loaded with less-than-pregnancy-friendly ingredients such as paraben preservatives and artificial fragrances, as well as botanicals and essential oils contraindicated in pregnancy.

NATURAL INGREDIENTS TO AVOID IN PREGNANCY

Caffeine
Retinols
Salicylic acid (also known as beta hydroxy acid)
Soy (may cause melasma)
Black henna
Gotu Kola
Aloe vera
Essential oils of:
Basil
Cedarwood
Cinnamon
Clary sage
Clove
Dill
Hyssop
Jasmine
Juniper
Lemongrass
Myrrh
Parsley
Rosemary
Oakmoss and treemoss

You can spend hours if not days researching pregnancy-safe skincare, but the easiest way to go is to make simple cleansers, creams, and stretch mark body serums yourself. Besides, essential oils have many beneficial effects and are safe when used in the right proportion.

Start with very gentle cleansing. Very simple, unscented castile soap will leave your skin clean and glowing without stripping away your natural protective barrier. For a toner, use green tea or witch hazel, especially if you are plagued with pregnancy acne. Sun creams with mineral protection of zinc oxide and titanium dioxide will protect your skin from uneven pigmentation called melasma, also known as the "mask of pregnancy." You can strengthen your skin's resilience to sun rays by taking antioxidant supplements with lycopene and lutein.

For nighttime care, make yourself a simple skin-nourishing oil with a lightweight base oil such as jojoba and a few drops of pregnancy-safe essential oils such tangerine, neroli, chamomile, lavender, frankincense, peppermint, ylang-ylang, eucalyptus, and tea tree oil—really great for pregnancy acne, but please discontinue its use during the last four weeks of pregnancy. You may have an individual, unique reaction to essential oils, while some of them may cause uterine contractions, which may lead to miscarriage.

Stretch marks are probably the most common skin concern in pregnancy. Nearly impossible to erase, they are preposterously easy to prevent. To help your skin stretch without tearing, massage 1 tablespoon of the following stretch mark body formula twice a day into your belly area—right from the moment your pregnancy test reveals the great news.

> **Stretch mark blend:** ½ cup olive oil (not necessarily extra virgin), ½ cup sunflower, ½ cup grapeseed, and 3 tablespoons castor seed oil. Shake well. These oils should ideally be organic. Keep the blend in a glass or polyethylene (plastic #2, also marked as PE) bottle. Avoid PET

(polyethylene terephthalate) bottles, as oils can
dissolve some of the plastic so that phthalate
would leach into the oil.

Minimizing phthalate exposure is important at any time of
your life, but during pregnancy you must avoid anything that can
contain plasticizer compounds. Phthalate exposure during pregnancy is linked to increased risk of allergy[132] and asthma,[133] penis
deformations in boys (hypospadias), testicular cancer and reduced
semen quality in men,[134] ADHD,[135] and hormonal disorders[136]
and obesity[137] later in life. Hormone-disrupting chemicals are
found in lots of everyday products including plastic bottles, metal
food cans (lined with epoxy resin), detergents, flame retardants,
food additives, toys, cosmetics, and pesticides.

While it's impossible to completely eliminate hormone-bending
chemicals from your life, take small steps by choosing mineral
water in glass rather than plastic bottles, or better yet, drinking
filtered tap water from BPA-free bottles. If you garden, switch to
natural pesticides and compost for soil fertilizing. Avoid conventional air fresheners, heavily scented laundry detergents and
house cleaning products, nonorganic scented candles, conventional perfumes, and any skincare that has been scented with
artificial fragrance. To add some olfactory spice to your life, find
an essential oil that pleases your senses (make sure it is safe for
use in pregnancy) and use it generously. Add it to the natural
dishwashing liquid, pop a few drops into the bucket of water when
you clean the floor, add to the detergent compartment when you
do the laundry, and to a bowl of water to place under the radiator
to moisten the air in your home.

As your body changes, you may notice your breasts sagging.
Bust-firming body oil is a little luxury that helps moisturize,
smooth, and firm up the bosom by boosting collagen and elastin
production. Here's a very simple recipe: Add 5 drops neroli essential oil, 5 drops ylang-ylang essential oil, and 5 drops frankincense essential oil to 150 mL (5 fl. oz.) sweet almond or grapeseed

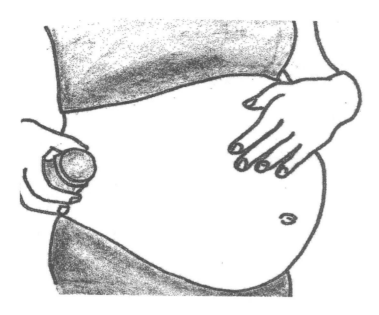

oil. Shake well and let stand for one day. I recommend using a glass bottle to store all body oils that contain essential oils.

To reap its full rewards, apply bust-firming lotions morning and night. Spread a teaspoon of oil from under the breasts to the base of the neck, avoiding the nipple area. You can also use it to massage the areas where you expect (or already have) stretch marks. Supporting underwear, yoga, and swimming are still the best bust-lifting methods around.

Your feet can become swollen and tired, especially toward the last three months of pregnancy. Always wear comfortable shoes, ideally made of non-tanned leather. When possible, wear shoes with special stimulating and massaging insoles, and walk barefoot frequently on grass or sand. To ease swollen ankles, try peppermint foot baths: brew a cup of very strong peppermint tea (3–4 packets per cup boiling water) and pour the infusion into a tub of tepid water. For added cooling effect, you can add a few drops of peppermint essential oil.

Foot exercises are also very useful to boost circulation and relieve tiredness:

1. Stretch your toes apart and close together (repeat 10 times);
2. Curl toes under, then extend (repeat 10 times);
3. Pinch the end of each toe between thumb and index finger;
4. Rotate the foot at ankle several times;
5. Stand on tiptoe for a few seconds or as long as you can, then relax (repeat 5 times).

You can do these exercises anytime, even in a car or while waiting for a doctor's appointment. And remember that smiling, stress-relieving relaxation, and great sleep will boost your pregnancy glow much better than any skincare in the world.

GORGEOUS HANDS NATURALLY

Anyone who multitasks—raising children, doing household chores, gardening, typing a lot—finds that an occasional slick of hand cream and maybe a weekly nail polish change would be the only ways to express gratitude to your fingers and hands for all the hard work they do.

To achieve healthy nails and smooth hands, you do not need to spend a fortune on gel extensions or salon paraffin wraps. Keeping your nails moisturized is one simple trick that will create the groomed, "just out from the salon" look at nearly zero cost. Nails are very porous and can become dehydrated just as easily as the skin can. Not surprisingly, oil is your nails' best friend. You can use any vegetable oil for this purpose or, if you like to experiment, you can add a few drops of chamomile or tea tree oil to the blend for antibacterial and healing properties. Massaging your nails and cuticles at least once a day before bed with vegetable oil will seal the moisture in, nourish the nail bed with fatty acids, and promote the circulation so that the nail grows strong and healthy.

Your nails respond to the quality of your diet. The nail plate is made up of several layers of keratin, which is the most abundant protein in our body. In strong nails, those layers are sealed together. But if your nails become weak and brittle—for example, after dealing with harsh detergents or when exposed to cold, dry air—those layers tend to break apart. According to traditional Chinese medicine principles, nail problems stem from an imbalance in gallbladder and liver function. I notice that with artichoke supplements, my nails and skin take an instant turn for better.

Peeling nails can also signal that your diet is lacking in linoleic acid. Simply adding a teaspoon of pure olive, coconut, or sunflower oil to your salads can prevent your nails from peeling.

Silica can also contribute to strong, smooth nails. Silica helps strengthen not only nails, skin, and hair but also other joints and ligaments in your body. Silica gels and supplements infused with the herb horsetail are widely available. Do not apply silica directly to your skin or nails, though, as inhaling silica microparticles can damage your lungs. Naturopaths recommend taking a silica supplement for three months and taking a break for one month before embarking on another course. Taking the break is important in any supplementation course for a number of reasons. First, science simply has no information on all the effects of long-term, high-dosage supplementation with vitamins or minerals. Second, some supplements, even the most benign ones, may accumulate in your tissues and potentially cause harm.

Thin, brittle, and easily broken nails are often the sign of iron deficiency. You can correct this problem by eating more green leafy vegetables, red meat, and eggs. Supplementing with biotin (a vitamin from the B group) also helps to improve the condition of brittle nails.

Constant water exposure can make nails dry and brittle, so if large, bulky rubber gloves aren't exactly your game, try neat surgical gloves from pharmacies—these days, you can buy them in latex-free and non-powdered versions. Gloves are essential for winter too, as they help protect the skin and nails from dehydration. Leather gloves with cashmere or silk lining are a luxury, but fleece gloves will shield your hands from elements just as well, if not as prettily.

NATURAL MANICURES FOR HEALTHY NAILS

Treat your hands with a natural manicure once a week. It takes only fifteen minutes of your time and is a great alternative to chemical-laden nail salons where you inhale acetone and formaldehyde vapors while being treated to "professional quality" nail products loaded with artificial dyes, fragrances, and preservatives.

To begin with, remove nail polish (if you wear it) with acetone-free polish remover such EDEN Natural Nail Varnish Remover (turn to Appendix C for more information). Then, rinse your nails with cold water to remove all traces of the chemicals.

Prepare a nail bath by immersing 2–3 packets of green or herbal teas in a bowl of very hot water. Allow the herbs to infuse while the water cools down, and when the water is warm, add 2–3 drops lavender, rosemary, or chamomile essential oil. Soak your fingertips in the water for five to seven minutes.

Rub your cuticles with a slice of lemon and allow the juice to sit on your fingertips for three to five minutes. Gently push your cuticles back with a wooden stick with a little cotton moistened with vegetable oil. Do not cut your cuticles. If there's a bit of overgrowth, you can gently file them off with a glass file.

File your nails in the desired shape using strokes, aiming from nail corners toward the center of the nail.

Instead of a paraffin treatment, the healing power of honey can be used for your weekly hand wrap. Fructose in honey acts as a natural antibacterial factor, which kills most types of bacteria, even those resilient to antibiotics. If the skin on your hands tends to crack—these cracks can be extremely painful when they occur around fingernails—cover your hands with honey whisked with an egg yolk, and cover with plastic gloves, then warm mittens. Leave the honey on your hands for at least thirty minutes or overnight, if you can, then rinse off and apply a hand cream or cuticle oil.

If you are not in the mood for nail polish, buff your nails and massage a little nail oil into the surface. If you do wear nail polish, choose toluene-free, formaldehyde-free brands such as Zoya or Scotch Naturals (for shopping suggestions, please check Appendix C). There are many mainstream brands that remove toxic nasties from their nail polishes, so it's worth checking the label of your familiar drugstore nail products in case they have turned for better. And when you paint your nails, stay near the open window if you can so that you don't inhale too much solvent vapors.

Chapter Twelve Quick Tips

1. **Shower with care: Choose detergent-free shower gels or** make your own body cleansers using castile soap, glycerine, plant oils, and essential oils.
2. Body oils are the skin's best moisturizers. **Blend your own body oils with base oils** and added essential oils to suit your current skin condition.
3. Skin brushing and natural scrubs keep your skin glowing all year round. **Brush your skin before every shower or a bath to beat cellulite** and keep your skin glowing and firm.
4. Cellulite serums cannot guarantee dimple-free skin: **Exercise, massage, regular fluid intake and fluid-flushing massaging oil with birch** are more reliable in your fight against cellulite.
5. **Natural tan supplements with carotenoids are safer and more reliable in your quest for a sunless tan** than tanning lotions loaded with potentially harmful ingredients.

6. Seawater and thalassotherapy **spa treatments can be easily replicated at home** for a fraction of a cost of salon treatments.

7. **Stretch marks, swollen feet, and pigmentation during pregnancy can be prevented** and eased with natural solutions such as oil blends, foot bathes, and mineral sunblocks.

8. **Eggs, silica, linoleic acid, and oils are your nails' best friends**—along with a natural manicure with green tea and.

9. Aluminum is carcinogenic, and present in all antiperspirants. **Opt for a natural alternative.**

THIRTEEN

Brilliantly Glowing Hair

Poetically called our "crowning glory," hair for many of us is the deepest misery as we struggle to add volume, straighten frizz, or add glisten to dull locks. We try to boost our confidence and self-esteem with a full-blown hair session in the morning, complete with a shampoo, hair mask, hair serum, blow dry, and possibly straightening. But how often can we manage to squeeze this indulgence into our mornings crammed with burnt toast, a malfunctioning coffee machine, a little one's sudden aversion to white stockings, lost keys, lost umbrellas, lost phones, and our lost temper, after all? No wonder that many of us adopt a no-fuss hairstyle routine: for long hair, a ponytail; for a bob, that "clean hair" flat look; and for super-short crop, well, the less you wash it, the better it looks—choppy and muddled. Can we find a holistic approach that won't rob us of a much-needed hour of sleep each morning?

Start with the condition of your hair. No matter how many silicones, vitamins, and essential oils you put on your hair, the trick will vanish at midnight, if not sooner. As with all parts of your body, true hair conditioning begins on your plate and in your cup. And on your pillow.

FEED YOUR HAIR

Eating well benefits your hair in general, but if you feel your hair could use an extra kick to help it grow faster or more thickly, then you should build your diet around hair-friendly nutrients. Strong hair begins in healthy skin of the scalp, so follow the same dietary recommendations I made for skin in earlier chapters, and boost your intake of hair-beautifying vitamins and antioxidants listed below. Fish, seaweed, nuts, seeds, legumes, dairy products, and cheese; all non-sweet, non-starchy vegetables such as peppers, avocados, cucumbers, asparagus, and aubergines; and lots of other brightly colored vegetables and fruit contain just the right amounts of naturallybalanced proteins, oils, fiber, vitamins, and minerals (most important, silica).

Our hair is built of keratin, which is a protein, so eating lots of good-quality proteins is vital for healthy hair. Fresh, minimally processed and preferably organic proteins for your hair come from lean meats and dairy, fish, eggs, nuts, seeds, pulses, and legumes. Brazil nuts, fish, shellfish, chicken, garlic, whole grains, and sunflower seeds also supply your hair with trace mineral selenium, an important antioxidant that not only wards off free radicals but also helps metabolize proteins so your hair and skin receive more nourishment and structural support.

Vitamin A is an essential antioxidant that helps restore healthy sebum flow in the scalp, and helps to relieve hair dryness, flakiness, and itchy scalp. Food sources include meat, milk, cheese, eggs, spinach, broccoli, cabbage, carrots, apricots, and peaches. Recommended daily dosage to improve your hair condition should be around 5,000 IU. Do not take more than 25,000 IU a day, as it can be extremely toxic and can cause hair loss as well as other serious health problems.

We already know how vital vitamin E is for the state of our skin, but it also helps maintain the healthy glow in our hair. This multitasking antioxidant improves blood circulation in the scalp and prevents the scalp from dehydration. All cold-pressed vegetable oils, seeds, and nuts, beans, and leafy green vegetables are good sources of vitamin E. To improve your hair condition and help prevent hair loss, aim for up to 400 IU vitamin E a day. Make sure to consult your medical practitioner if you suffer from high blood pressure, as this vitamin may not be suitable for you. Instead, infuse your scalp with vitamin E by applying weekly warm oil treatments (see below for details on oil treatments).

Biotin stimulates keratin production so that hair becomes stronger and maintains its natural color. Biotin naturally contains in brewer's yeast, whole grains, egg yolks, liver, and dairy products. If you decide to supplement with biotin, aim for 150–300 mcg a day.

Niacin, also known as vitamin B3, maintains good blood circulation in the scalp so your hair receives fresh oxygen and nutrients. Apart from brewer's yeast, niacin is found in wheat germ, fish, chicken, turkey, and meat. If you choose to supplement with niacin, take up to 15 mg a day. Vitamins of the B group are best taken as a complex because all of them are very helpful for the skin and hair.

Essential fatty acids (EFAs) help restore hair luster and manageability. By maintaining a steady flow of sebum, EFAs relieve hair dryness and itchy, flaking scalp, which many people mistake for dandruff. Instead of reaching for an antidandruff shampoo, pop a fish or starflower (borage) oil capsule after meals three times a day and make weekly warm oil treatments with hemp seed oil.

Zinc helps restore healthy hormonal levels. Sometimes the abundance in male hormone testosterone leads to hair loss and even pattern baldness in women. Zinc regulates testosterone levels and at the same time improves your immune response so that your scalp becomes less disturbed by elements or aggressive hairstyling. Rich food sources of zinc include oysters, red meats, poultry, liver, brewer's yeast, wheat germ, pumpkin seeds, mussels, shrimps, egg yolks, nuts, and various soy products. Better supplements of zinc should contain zinc gluconate, zinc arginate, or zinc citrate, which are better absorbed by the body. In addition to a healthy diet, supplementing your diet with a vitamin B complex, essential fatty acids, and glow-boosting vitamins C and E will make a very noticeable change for better in your hair's condition. Taking a rich multivitamin pill with a complete list of essential minerals is also helpful. Check with your doctor before taking any supplements, as this may have adverse effects on your overall health.

It takes about a month or so for the hair to absorb the hair vitamins and get into the system. You should start seeing your hair grow at a rate of an inch per month.

Emotional stress has a direct effect on the condition of your hair. Stress makes the muscles of your neck and head become stiff and tense, which reduces the blood flow to the scalp. To reduce tension, you can try yoga, meditation, or head and neck massage offered at very affordable prices in many spas and salons. I found that my stress-triggered hair loss has greatly diminished after a few sessions of acupuncture, which I initially hoped would deal with headaches and tinnitus. These deeply relaxing sessions helped my head all over, from my brain down to my split ends!

SHAMPOO WITH CARE

Did you know your hair needs a full twenty-four hours to restore its natural balance after a shampoo? If you treat your hair to a portion of bubbles every day, chances are, you do not allow the scalp to saturate the hair shaft with enough oil, as all of the oil will be used to moisturize the scalp until the next detergent attack. As a result, you set your hair up for dryness and breakage. To shampoo your hair really well, try these tips:

1. Gently brush your hair before shampooing to help the cleansing agent penetrate between every strand.
2. Massage the shampoo well into the scalp, and then leave it on to penetrate for a whole minute to reap full benefits of the shampoo. (More on what shampoo to use below.)
3. Use warm or lukewarm water for shampooing, and rinse with cooler water to close the hair shaft and boost the shine.
4. Rinse well, keeping water running through your hair longer than you think you need. Shampoo residue can make your hair dull and dry.

There seems to be an avalanche of organic shampoos available, but a closer look at the ingredients list reveals that not all of them are as natural as the manufacturer wants us to believe. Common chemicals "sneaking in" most so-called organic hair cleansers include diethanolamine (DEA), various petrochemicals identified as PEG and propylene glycol, polyquaterniums, phenoxyethanol, ethylhexyl glycerine, methylisothiazolinone, DMDM hydantoin, and artificial fragrances. The biggest no-no to watch out for is sodium laureth sulfate, which is a harsh detergent that not only leaves hair brittle and the scalp taut, but is also harmful for the environment.

Some of my favorite all-natural shampoos include Burt's Bees Very Volumizing Shampoo, Pomegranate and Soy; California Baby Shampoo & Bodywash in Calendula; and a cooling Desert Essence Tea Tree Replenishing Shampoo with Peppermint and Yucca—great for summertime.

Making your own shampoo at home is quite easy. All you need is some natural olive soap and glycerine. Measure 120 mL (4 fl. oz.) castile soap in a bottle; Add 1 tablespoon glycerine, and 1 tablespoon of an oil of your choice. Here are some combinations that you can add to the castile soap and glycerine to further customize to your liking:

Dry, brittle hair: 2 tablespoons extra virgin olive oil, 4 drops peppermint, and 3 drops myrrh essential oils.

Dandruff: 1 tablespoon jojoba oil, 10 drops lavender, 5 drops ylang-ylang and 5 drops tea tree essential oils.

Hair loss: 1 tablespoon castor seed oil, 5 drops clary sage, and 10 drops rosemary essential oils.

Hair growth: 1 tablespoon extra-virgin olive oil, 5 drops basil, and 10 drops rosemary essential oils.

Oily scalp: 1 teaspoon jojoba oil, 10 drops geranium, and 10 drops tea tree essential oils. You can also add a good teaspoon of white or green clay to the shampoo—it will absorb excess oil without overdrying.

Itchy scalp: 2 tablespoons grapeseed oil, 10 drops rose otto, and 5 drops lavender essential oils.

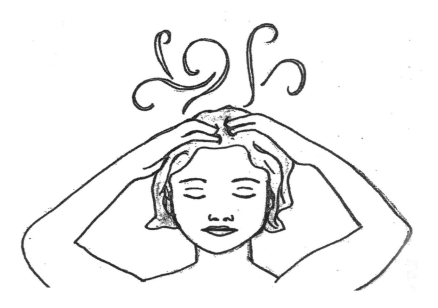

Most experts recommend shampooing every other day, but if you just cannot live with unwashed hair, try this Apple Cider Vinegar Rinse in place of a regular shampoo: Add 2 tablespoons apple cider vinegar to a cupful water and rinse your hair. Result: dazzling glow, no chemicals involved. I encourage you to prepare a large bottle of this rinse, as it doesn't go stale or weak, and experiment with essential oils for natural hair fragrance and scalp benefit. However, note that blondes should never use apple cider vinegar.

Dry shampoos are becoming increasingly popular as they help skip the daily dose of detergents and save time too, especially if you are in a hurry and not in a mood for a shampoo (or if you simply love the hairstyle and want to prolong it for one more day).

Most dry shampoos contain talc, which may be harmful for your health if you accidentally inhale too much. You can easily make your own natural dry shampoo by mixing 1 cup each of cornstarch, white clay, and baking soda. You can also add a few drops of your favorite essential oil to the blend. Transfer the mixture to a sifter jar and pour 1 tablespoon of mixture into your hand. Make sure your hands are clean and cream free. Now rub your hands together to spread the powder, and start rubbing it into your locks starting at roots to absorb any oil. It's best to apply dry shampoo over a sink because it can be quite messy. Scrunch and toss your hair until all powder disappears. This trick can restore bounce in hat-flattened hair during the winter. You can also use it in the evening to wake up in the morning to full, bouncy hair. Dry shampoos can leave your hair a little dull, so you can restore shine with a careful swipe of shine-enhancing serum or argan oil—but limit its use on hair ends only, otherwise your hair will end up looking greasy *and* dull.

Conditioner for your hair is the same as a moisturizer for your skin; in other words, it is essential, especially if your hair has been chemically treated, colored, or baked under the midday sun recently. Carefully squeeze excess water from your hair and apply a generous portion of the conditioner of your choice. Most conventional hair conditioners have very similar formulas loaded with silicones, polyquaterniums, and occasionally protein. All of these can irritate your scalp and cause even more problems than you were trying to solve. Here are some really simple all-natural conditioner ideas that you can use without risk of irritation, itchiness, or dryness:

Whole eggs: Rich in lecithin and protein, eggs add shine and strength to normal to oily hair. Rub in gently until the egg foams, leave on for one minute, and rinse off.

Coconut milk: Ideal for all hair types but especially dry hair. Apply straight from the container and rinse after a minute or two.

Jojoba oil: Don't dread the word "oil," as it won't make your hair flat or limp. A weekly hot oil pack with jojoba oil helps prevent and treat dandruff and itchy scalp. To treat your hair with oil, rub 2–3 tablespoons of oil (depending on your hair length) into your dry, unwashed hair, starting at roots, and cover it first with plastic cap and then with a towel. Walk around for fifteen to twenty minutes, then shampoo as usual.

Rye bread and water: Soak 2–3 slices of rye bread (remove the crust) in 1 cup water, mash to achieve a custard-like consistency, and apply to your hair, massaging deeply into the scalp. Leave on for two to three minutes, then rinse off.

Plain yogurt: Great for all hair types but especially for dull, limp hair. Apply straight from the package, leave on the hair for one or two minutes, then rinse off.

Applesauce: Apply to your hair after washing to reveal gorgeous glow and less dandruff and itchiness after just one application.

Avocado and olive oil: Mash 1 avocado with 1 tablespoon of olive oil to make a deeply nourishing spread for your hair. Apply to your hair, then cover with a plastic cap and a towel to keep hair warm, and to improve the penetration of these beneficial ingredients.

Honey and egg hair mask: Combine ½ cup runny honey with 1 egg yolk and 1 tablespoon brandy (optional). Whisk well and apply to your hair, massaging well into the roots. Cover up with a plastic bonnet and a towel so your hair remains warm. Rinse off.

Honey and avocado hair mask: This mask restores brilliant glow in the hair. Combine ½ cup honey or more, depending on your hair length, and add ½ mashed avocado. Whisk till creamy and apply to your hair, focusing on split ends, if you have any. Rinse off after thirty minutes. Enjoy the glow!

NATURAL HAIR TREATMENTS

Hair is probably the last organ to benefit from any nutritional boost, so it is necessary to nourish it not just from the inside out, but also from the outside in. Once a week (or twice if your hair is very damaged and brittle) give your hair an extra-nourishing oil treatment. Choose argan, olive, or castor seed oil if you've noticed you are losing more hair than usual—or combine the oils until you find the blend that makes your hair look and feel spectacular. Heat the oils slightly in a pan, then shampoo and towel-dry your hair. Comb the hair carefully with a wide-tooth comb, then carefully saturate your hair with the oil and again run the comb through your hair to evenly distribute. Cover your head with a plastic shower cap or vinyl-free cling wrap and wrap a towel over your head to keep the hair warm.

As the oil penetrates each and every hair strand and your

scalp, you can try a very simple scalp massage. It helps improve blood circulation and relieve tension, thus helping to nourish the hair follicles with fresh oxygen and nutrients. Scalp massage is especially beneficial if you suffer from a dry, flaking scalp; seborrhoea (a skin condition that makes your scalp itchy, red, and covered with pimples); or if you are concerned about hair loss. There are no set rules for scalp massage other than it should be done with firm pressing movements and last for three minutes or more. Rub, press, and glide your fingertips across your scalp and down to the temples, as long as it feels good and doesn't scratch or pull your hair. Scalp massage, invokes an immense sense of relaxation and brings a lovely glow to your skin. After eight to ten minutes, shampoo your hair again and go on styling as usual.

HEALTHY SCALP

Glowing, strong hair starts with a healthy scalp. Ironically, the hair as we see it is made of dead, flattened keratin cells, and only a tiny part hiding underneath the scalp is living and reproducing. Hair grows from a dermal papilla hiding in a hair follicle nourished by blood vessels. To maintain healthy growth, cells in papilla must receive enough nutrients and oxygen from surrounding dermal tissue. Hair-forming cells are one of the fastest-dividing in the human body, so if you notice change for worse in your hair condition, it's a clear sign that your general health has taken change for worse too.

To nourish the scalp, prepare a purée of 2 apricots and 1 ripe peach by mashing them with a fork or blending in a food processor. Apply to clean, towel-dried hair, leave for eight to ten minutes, and rinse off. You hair will be very shiny and bouncy. Stress, hormonal imbalance, certain medications, and even fever can dry out the scalp and make it less able to nourish and support hair follicles. Following a healthy diet with ample amounts of essential fatty acids, zinc, iron, copper, and iodine will maintain healthy hair growth and help prevent scalp problems such as dandruff and seborrhea.

TAKING CARE OF COLORED HAIR

For those of us who color our hair, even if we are happy with our current color, it may still require regular upkeep, such as monthly colorings. Conventional hair dyes contain an untold number of toxic ingredients that have only been partially studied for short- and long-term safety for animals, and never for humans. To avoid contaminating your body and setting yourself up for higher risk of cancer, give natural hair dyes a try.

Blondes

Hair shades carry a lot of meaning. For instance, we all know that blondes have more fun, right? Perhaps we do, since hair-care product companies estimate that in the United States, 40 percent of women who color their hair choose blond shades.[138] Some researchers say blond hair suggests a childlike appearance, as many newborns have very light hair that darkens with age. Blond is probably the only color that gets better with age, as gray strands can turn into silvery highlights in the hands of a skilled colorist. Here are simple home recipes that will infuse your blond locks with a lovely glow yet leave no traces of toxins in your system:

> **Lemon and Yogurt Glow Booster**: Alpha hydroxy acids in lemon juice restore shine and lightly exfoliate the scalp, while yogurt does the same trick with lactic acid, and adds proteins for hair nourishment. Combine 1 small tub (4 oz.) of plain yogurt with the juice of a half or whole lemon, depending on your hair length and volume. Leave on for five to ten minutes, then rinse off.
>
> **Potato and Applesauce Mask**: Raw potatoes contain the lightening enzyme catecholase, which not

only helps erase under-eye circles, but also lightens your hair. Grate one raw potato and squeeze the juice from the pulp. Add up to 1 cup of applesauce to the potato juice and stir well. Add cornstarch if the mask is too runny. Apply the mask on towel-dried hair and leave for at least ten minutes. Rinse and gasp in amusement as you see your hair lightened and brightened without any chemicals.
Avocado and Egg Yolk: While it is great for all hair types and colors, this simple mask is especially good for blond hair, as it tends to be more porous and therefore can become limp and flat with heavy oil treatments. Avocado supplies proteins and lightweight fatty acids, while egg yolk strengthens the hair with lecithin and proteins. Simply mash 1 avocado with 1 egg yolk and make a face lifting mask with the egg white. Apply the hair pack and keep covered with a plastic shower cap for ten minutes or as long as you can, then rinse off.

Brunettes

Brunette hair color is so low maintenance, it leaves natural brunettes a lot more time for fun while blondes are busy fussing with outgrown roots. I may convert to blonde when silver hairs on my head outnumber dark brown ones. But for the time being, I enjoy my natural no-nonsense chocolate brown color, which I can enhance with a lightly diluted infusion of black henna as a rinse, or strongly brewed black tea or coffee for shine and color maintenance.

Black tea is a wholesome yet inexpensive hair treatment. Black tea is rich in catechins, tannins, amino acids, vitamins, minerals, and essential oils. Prepare a very strong black tea infusion (1 cup black tea leaves per 3 cups water) by boiling loose tea with water for two or three minutes and then letting it steep and cool down for an hour. Rinse your hair after shampooing. This solution also works for blond hair whose owners decided to go a few shades darker without any of the risks associated with conventional hair dyes. For best results, leave black tea on your hair for ten minutes, or until your hair begins to dry naturally. Rinse and style as you prefer.

Henna-based dark and coppery shades require long-term commitment, as you cannot switch from henna to chemicals and vice versa. Still, if you plan to stay in your color family and do not plan dramatic color changes, henna is worth the effort. Today you can find lots of henna-based hair colors offered by such brands as Light Mountain, LUSH, Tints of Nature, and Rainbow Research. Even blondes can try henna now! If you are used to thoughtfully packaged conventional hair dye kits where all you need to do is connect, click, and squeeze, well, henna kits are not as sophisticated. You will need to do some pouring, mixing, and applying with a brush. If you welcome some golden hue to your hair tone, do not cover your hair with a cling film. If you want exact color results, top the henna "helm" on your head with a plastic film and cover it with a towel to keep it warm.

Now you must entertain yourself for one or two hours while the henna works its magic. Here is some time for a bit of yoga, meditation, or, you can finally sort that cupboard in your bedroom, cook a few batches of curry and freeze them, and (how could I forget) do your mani-pedi. Trust me, the results are well worth the wait. Regardless of the henna blend you choose, your hair will become incredibly radiant, less prone to falling out, and overall a lot healthier.

Dark-tinted hair is naturally more resilient to the elements, and therefore can withstand a little apple cider or white wine vinegar diluted in proportion 1 part vinegar to 4 parts water as a rinse. Vinegars act as gentle oxidizers working to break apart the melanin molecules inside the hair shaft, thus bleaching the hair. You can also try this rinse instead of a daily shampoo, if you have not used too many styling products.

Redheads

Speaking of color maintenance, redheads perhaps have the most fun spending the least time fussing about their hair being shiny or resilient. I have never seen a redhead with dull hair full of split ends! But still, that gorgeous sunny mane will benefit from regular shine-enhancing treatments. For this purpose, fruit juices make the easiest, most natural yet immensely effective hair rinses. Carrot juice is the obvious choice, and for a good reason, as it not only colors but also nourishes the scalp with beta-carotene. Citrus juices work their shine-boosting magic, and cranberry deepens the golden hue while imparting a lovely glow to auburn locks. Lighter shades of the redhead family would also benefit from a chamomile rinse: place 3–4 packets of chamomile tea or 1 cup dried chamomile flowers in 2 cups boiling water, infuse for five minutes, cool down, strain, and stream through your hair (no need to rinse out). Darker shades of copper and chestnut will love strongly brewed rooibos tea as a hair rinse after shampooing.

NATURAL HELP FOR HAIR LOSS

We normally shed somewhere between fifty and one hundred hairs every day, but nutritional deficiencies such as lack of protein or iron, ongoing emotional or physical stress, dandruff or eczema, and hormonal changes can all cause your hair to leave its "habitual residence" at a quicker pace, more than a few hundred a day. A recent study found other hidden causes of hair loss in women: multiple marriages, longer sleep duration, higher severity of stress, smoking history, lack of exercise, history of diabetes mellitus, polycystic ovarian syndrome, and hypertension.[139] Women are particularly prone to hair loss during times of profound hormonal changes, for example, when they start or stop taking a contraceptive pill or during pregnancy or menopause.

There are many traps and natural disasters that threaten our path to a glowing, strong mane of hair. Thankfully, there are ways to preserve your crowning glory.

Stress can be a major hair scavenger. It has been estimated that physical stress, such as childbirth, can trigger dramatic yet (thanks!) temporary hair loss of up to 50 percent. Thinning hair can be due to a lack of iron, so if your hair loss is accompanied with fatigue, pale skin, headaches, sore tongue, brittle nails, and muscle cramps, you may be well on your way to iron deficiency. Load up on lean red meat, beef and chicken liver, lentils, soybeans, fortified oatmeal, spinach, and green leafy vegetables. An underactive thyroid can also be a cause for hair loss. Foods rich in iodine, such as haddock or cod, can help restore balance, but you must check with your health practitioner to rule out any thyroid diseases.

Hair loss may also be due to poor circulation. Scalp massage with castor seed oil is a very potent, traditional remedy for hair loss, so try to pair a castor oil scalp massage with meditation or yoga. Don't forget to rub the remaining castor oil into your lashes or eyebrows to help them grow strong. Do not believe in the myth (it's very common in hair salons) that vitamins rubbed into hair or scalp will stop your hair loss. The only way vitamins can benefit your hair is through balanced diet and careful supplementation.

Handle your thinning hair with care: avoid brushing it too vigorously; steer clear from appliances that pull, scorch, or twist the hair; and ideally leave the hair to dry naturally.

Add good proteins, essential fatty acids, and calcium to your diet; sleep the recommended seven hours at least; and examine your lifestyle for any "hair enemies" such as stress, a "fast-food" diet, too much styling, harsh hair dyes, chlorinated water, or excessive sun exposure without a hat.

When all fails, read these words by a woman whose hair length barely reached two inches, yet who was (and is) the loveliest, most sincere beauty icon of all time: "The beauty of a woman must be seen from in her eyes, because that is the doorway to her heart, the place where love resides."

Thank you, Audrey Hepburn!

Chapter Thirteen Quick Tips

1. **Prepare your own shampoo** by combining plant oils, glycerine, and essential oils with a basic castile soap. If your scalp is oily or flaking, you can add a few teaspoons of clay to the shampoo so it becomes oil absorbing.

2. **Coconut milk, fruit and vegetable juices, and apple cider vinegar make wonderful and easy hair conditioners.** You can splash your hair with juices straight from the container. Dilute apple cider vinegar in plain water for gloss-boosting rinse or in chamomile tea if you want to lighten your locks.

3. Vitamins A, B, C, and E, as well as proteins and zinc, are essential for healthy hair growth. If you show signs of deficiency, such as shedding too much hair, **boost iron-rich foods, and consider supplementing with iron as you might be iron deficient—** but please consult with your health provider first.

4. **Oil treatments and hair masks are excellent for all hair types**, as they help condition the hair and revitalize the scalp.

5. **Colored hair can be revived** with homemade colorants containing yogurt, chamomile, coffee, carrots, or cocoa.

CONCLUSION

If there's one lesson you decide to learn from this book, make it this: you are responsible for your beauty. Period. You are the only person who can decide which beauty products work for you. Only after you start being proactive about your looks instead of reacting to the newest ad, the newest fad diet, the newest "runway look," only then you will be able to make independent decisions when it comes to your skincare, makeup, and general well-being that will enhance your beauty, inside and out

Another idea worth sinking in: looking good has nothing to do with spending lots of money. You may need to adjust your mind-set, and move away from media-induced constant self-doubt, self-punishment, and self-belittlement. We have all seen horrible photos of expensive cosmetic surgeries that have gone wrong'. Sleeping well, learning to relax, eating antioxidant-rich foods, and drinking lots of water may easily replace the immediate need of antiwrinkle creams. Relieving stress and avoiding certain food groups in your diet may help erase blemishes without potentially toxic antibiotics or retinoids. Having a pet does wonders to your cellulite (hello, morning walks!) and self-esteem (hello, licking tongues, wagging tails, and adoring eyes!). Stress relief and dietary adjustments will strengthen your hair better than any pill, and a realistic, positive outlook toward aging will allow you to see your true beauty, which stands the test of time.

If you believe that science holds the answer for your beauty woes, think of the parabens and heavy metals that come with many commercial products and supposed beauty cures. Ask any dermatologist when you go for a yearly check-up of your moles and freckles, what she thinks of a whitening cream that contains mercury? Most likely, she will strongly advise you against its use (if she insists that you try such cream, you'd better run, not walk, away from that doctor). Twenty years ago mercury bleaching creams were widely recommended. Not a single dermatologist would question their safety. Today, mercury in cosmetics is banned worldwide. A whole new list of substances, such as parabens, lead, and phthalates, deserve a similar ban. I hope you will proactively rid your shelves of products with dangerous ingredients, before the official ban wipes them off store shelves. Pass on buying anything that has proved to be carcinogenic even in animal studies. That's right, humans are not rodents. But then again, DNA is DNA. If a substance damages a living creature's DNA and causes it to mutate or die altogether, there's a very high chance it will mess up human cells too.

Next time you reach for that pretty bottle, I hope that reading this book will cause you to stop for a second, read the list of ingredients, and ask yourself: Would I eat any of this? Let this question linger for a moment. Then close your wallet, head on to that humble health food store, and grab an unpretentious bottle of herbal body and hair wash. Better yet, grab a bottle of olive oil soap, some essential oils, and some glycerine. Spend two minutes blending them all together. Your hair will be just as clean, and much healthier, and you may sleep a little better, and live a little longer.

Your common sense is your best guide to sorting through the beauty myths, fads, and hype. Remember that the cosmetic industry spends billions of dollars each year to sell you one myth or another. Many of the so-called organic products only give you a sense of safety without being truly natural and safe. Spend a second or two scanning the ingredient list and refuse to buy anything that does not fit your idea of truly pure and natural beauty product.

Set yourself apart from the rest by letting the natural glow of your beauty shine through the artificials our life is filled with. Adopt and nurture a confident, self-reliant, and positive state of mind. After all, your life belongs to you, and you only, not to the smart marketers and cleverly Photoshopped models who make you feel inferior in order to promote snake oil packed in a fancy designer bottle. By making a commitment to natural beauty, you rid your life of synthetic junk and artificial, fake claims. Instead, you fill your life with genuine, priceless things that really matter: a good night's sleep, a happy smile after twenty minutes of meditation, a gulp of a delicious smoothie made of fresh watermelon and orange, a swish of clean hair free of silicone junk, and glowing skin after a vigorous body rub and a dot of olive oil lovingly massaged in.

Happy mind + clean diet + pure skin = the glow of holistic beauty.

Keep this equation in your heart and mind, and rejoice in the joys of treating yourself with the love and respect you deserve!

APPENDIX A

100 Toxic Ingredients Found in Beauty Products

This is an updated and revised list of toxic synthetic and natural ingredients currently used in skincare, hair care, makeup, and fragrances. Many of them are banned for use in the United States, Canada, or European Union but may still be found in your cosmetics. Refer to this list anytime you consider buying a beauty product and check your beauty stash for the presence of these nasties. Minimize your exposure to these chemicals, and if possible completely eliminate them from your beauty routine.

5-BROMO-5-NITRO-1,3 DIOXANE: found in sunblocks and bath products, this toxic preservative may be contaminated with carcinogenic dioxane and nitrosamines.

ALUMINUM CHLORIDE/OXY-CHLORIDE/HYDROCHLORIDE/STARCH: strong human neurotoxicant; causes irritation of eyes, skin, and lungs; endocrine disruptor; linked to Alzheimer's disease and breast cancer; causes birth disorders in animals; endocrine disruptor linked to breast cancer and Alzheimer's disease; aluminum compounds are neurotoxic to humans.

AMMONIUM LAURETH SULFATE: linked to skin irritation, water

contaminant, may be contaminated with carcinogen 1,4-dioxane.

AMMONIUM PERSULFATE: found in hair dyes, it is a strong human skin irritant and immune system suppresant; for these reasons it is restricted for use in cosmetics.

BENZALKONIUM CHLORIDE: affects the immune system, and is a lung and skin toxicant; can trigger asthma; restricted in Canada and Japan

BENZOCAINE: this sunblock ingredient and topical numbing agent has a proven effect of whole body toxicity and immune system damage.

BENZYL ALCOHOL: strong neurotoxicant; can cause allergic reaction in lungs; causes itching, burning, scaling, hives, and blistering of skin; caused liver damage, coma, and death in animals.

BENZYL SALICYLATE: this fragrance component and UV absorber is associated with allergies and contact dermatitis.

BORIC ACID: strong reproductive toxin; potent endocrine disruptor; unsafe for use on infant, injured, or damaged skin;

causes death and birth defects in animals; banned in Canada and Japan.

BRONOPOL (2-bromo-2-nitro-propane-1,3-diol): one of the strongest lung and skin toxicants; endocrine disruptor; forms carcinogenic nitrosamine; causes allergic contact dermatitis environmental contaminant; poisonous to wildlife.

BUTYLATED HYDROXYANISOLE (BHA): this chemical is a human carcinogen; caused brain and liver tumors in animals at low doses; endocrine disruptor; causes allergic contact dermatitis and skin depigmentation; banned in European Union; persistent environmental toxin.

BUTYLATED HYDROXYTOLUENE (BHT): common preservative in food and skincare, it is a known endocrine disruptor, and a skin and lung toxicant at low doses; causes death, liver and stomach cancers, thrombosis, fibrosis, liver and brain damage in animals; strong skin and eye irritant.

BUTYLENE GLYCOL: this solvent and thickener is a proven skin, lung, and eye irritant; environmental toxin.

BUTYLPARABEN: skin and eye irritant; endocrine disruptor linked to breast and ovarian cancer; environmental contaminant.

CADE (*Juniperus Oxycedrus*): extract or wood tar of this plant is a human neurotoxicant and strong skin irritant. It is classified as expected to be toxic or harmful. Found in organic creams.

CALCIUM FLUORIDE: neurotoxic to humans; leads to bone weakness; causes birth abnormalities and depression in animals.

CETEARETH (followed by numbers): unsafe for use on broken skin; eye and lung irritant; may be contaminated with 1,4-dioxane.

CETRIMONIUM CHLORIDE: skin and eye sensitizer that can include itching, burning, scaling, hives, and blistering; caused cell mutations in animal studies.

CHLOROACETAMIDE: strong skin, eye, and lung irritant; toxic if inhaled; causes paralysis, goiter, and birth defects in animals; banned in Canada.

CINNAMAL: this fragrance component is a known immune system toxicant and skin irritant. It is restricted for use in leave-on beauty products.

COAL TAR: proven human carcinogen; causes lung and urinary tract cancer; potent skin irritant; causes multiple cancers in animals; banned in most countries including Canada and European Union; still used in antidandruff shampoos in the United States.

COCAMIDE DEA (ethanolamide of coconut acid): strong human skin toxicant and suspected carcinogen; causes irritation of skin, eyes, and lungs in humans; causes liver and bladder cancer in animals.

D&C RED 30 LAKE: colorant which is a strong nervous system toxicant; as an aluminum compound, disrupts endocrine system and linked to breast and ovarian cancer; persistent wildlife contaminant.

D&C VIOLET 2: coal tar dye; skin and eye irritant; long-term use of coal tar hair dye linked to bladder cancer.

DIBUTYL PHTHALATE: neurotoxicant, linked to impaired fertility and urinary abnormalities, linked to breast and ovarian cancers, contaminates wildlife.

DIETHANOLAMINE (DEA): linked to brain abnormalities in animals; may be contaminated with carcinogen 1,4-dioxane.

DIMETICONE (dimethicone): petroleum derivative, environmental toxicant.

DMDM HYDANTOIN: contains carcinogenic FORMALDEHYDE; skin, eye, and lung irritant; environmental toxicant.

ELECAMPANE (inula helenium) EXTRACT: fragrance component banned as unsafe in European Union based on strong evidence of human neurotoxicity.

ETHYLPARABEN: skin and eye irritant; endocrine disruptor linked to breast and ovarian cancer; environmental contaminant.

FD&C BLUE 1: derived from coal tar; linked to allergies and hyperactivity disorders.

FD&C GREEN 3: linked to sarcomas and bone marrow hyperplasia in animals; not studied for safety in humans; prohibited in European Union.

FD&C YELLOW 5: causes severe allergic and intolerance reactions, especially among asthmatics and those with an aspirin intolerance; linked to thyroid tumors, chromosomal damage, hives, and hyperactivity in humans.

FD&C YELLOW 6: human skin and eye irritant; caused coma, convulsions, testicular damage, and changes in leucocytes in animals; cannot be used in eye cosmetics.

FIG (Ficus carica): immune system toxin; cannot be used as fragrance ingredient due to potential carcinogenicity; banned in European Union; allowed in the United States as fragrance ingredient in shampoos and body washes.

FORMALDEHYDE: known human carcinogen linked to leukemia; pancreatic, skin, liver, and lung cancer; strong skin, eye, and lung irritant; irritates human liver (causes cirrhosis), stomach, kidneys, and bladder; can cause skin burns; triggers asthma; hazardous air pollutant; environmental toxin; banned in Canada and Japan; determined as safe for use in cosmetics in the United States.

GLUTARAL: known as Cidex, this preservative is a skin and immune system toxicant. Found in soaps, moisturizers and hair conditioners.

GLYCERYL ROSINATE: this skin conditioner is also a known strong skin irritant.

HYDROABIETYL ALCOHOL: this fragrance compound is a known skin and immune system toxicant; restricted for use in cosmetics.

HYDROGENATED COTTONSEED OIL: may be contaminated with mercury, lead, arsenic, and pesticides unless certified organic.

HYDROQUINONE: eye, lung, and nervous system toxin; can cause itching, burning, scaling, hives, and blistering of skin; suspected liver and stomach carcinogen; causes liver cancer, DNA and ovary mutations in animals; restricted in Canada.

IMIDAZOLIDINYL UREA (Uric Acid): can cause itching, burning, scaling, hives, and blistering of skin

IODOPROPYNYL BUTYLCARBAMATE: contains DIETHANOLAMINE; can affect thyroid function; gastrointestinal or liver toxicant; cannot be used in aerosols; causes allergic contact dermatitis; restricted in Japan.

ISOPARAFFIN: petroleum derivative; environmental toxin; mildly irritating; produced kidney damage in animals; not carcinogenic in humans.

ISOPROPYL ALCOHOL (SD-40): human neurotoxin; skin, eye, and lung irritant; vapors cause drowsiness and dizziness; causes skin dehydration, may promote brown spots and premature aging of skin; petroleum derivative.

LACTIC ACID: strong skin and eye irritant; can cause skin burns; causes changes in liver, brain, and blood in animals; caused mutations and birth defects in animals; restricted in Canada.

LANOLIN: strong skin irritant and toxicant; can cause allergic reaction in the lungs; may be contaminated with pesticides absorbed by sheep wool.

LAURETH-7: petrochemical that may be contaminated with carcinogen 1,4-dioxane.

LEAD ACETATE: possible human carcinogen and neurotoxin;

skin and eye irritant; environmental toxin; banned in European Union.

LECITHIN: if not from plant origin, can irritate lungs in aerosol form; a potent asthma trigger; forms carcinogenic nitrosamine compounds if mixed with nitrosating agents.

MANGANESE SULFATE: strong human neurotoxin; harmful during prolonged exposure or inhalation; causes convulsions, DNA mutations, and protein loss in animals; toxic to wildlife.

METHENAMINE: this preservative is a strong human neurotoxin, immune system toxicant, and skin irritant banned for use in cosmetics. Can be found in shampoos, conditioners, and body powders.

METHYL CELLOSOLVE: this chemical is restricted for use in cosmetics as it is a known human developmental toxicant and neurotoxin. Can be found in eye creams, antiaging creams, and face moisturizers.

METHYL METHACRYLATE: strong neurotoxin; strong eye and lung irritant; causes asthma and skin burns; causes cancer and stomach bleeding in animals;

hazardous air pollutant; banned in Canada and recently in the United States.

METHYLDIBROMO GLUTARONITRILE: this preservative is a strong skin and immune system toxicant; found in sunscreen, moisturizers and body wash.

METHYLPARABEN: skin and eye irritant; endocrine disruptor linked to breast and ovarian cancer; environmental contaminant.

MINERAL OIL (liquid petrolatum): linked to blood and skin cancer formations in animals; eye and skin irritant; derived from petroleum; nonbiodegradable environmental toxin.

NAPHTHOL: this hair dye is a strong skin and lung irritant; potential carcinogen.

NONOXYNOL (ethoxylated alkyl phenol): endocrine disruptor; skin and lung irritant; caused liver damage in animals; may be contaminated with 1,4-dioxane.

OCTOXYNOL (10, 11, 13, 40): strong skin and eye toxin that can cause itching, burning, scaling, hives, and blistering of skin; may contain carcinogen

1,4-dioxane; caused cancer of reproductive organs in animals.

ONOETHANOLAMINE (MEA): skin and eye irritant at low doses, can be irritating to the respiratory tract.

OXYBENZONE (benzophenone-4): strong photoallergen, endocrine disruptor; produces free radicals that can increase skin aging; environmental toxicant.

PADIMATE O (octyl dimethyl PABA/PABA ester): has estrogenic activity; releases free radicals that damages DNA when exposed to sunlight; causes allergic reactions and photoallergenic dermatitis; restricted in Japan.

P-AMINOPHENOL: common hair dye ingredient which is a human immune system and skin toxicant; possible mutagen; environmental toxin.

PARA AMINO BENZONIC ACID (PABA): causes allergic dermatitis and photosensitivity; produces free radicals that cause mutations, lead to cell death, and may be implicated in cardiovascular disease; causes changes in blood components and muscle weakness in animals; banned in Canada.

PARAFFIN (*Parrafinum liquidum*): petrochemical bleached with carcinogen acrolyn; releases carcinogens benzene and toluene upon heating; caused kidney or renal system tumors in animals; environmental toxin.

PEG-40 CASTOR OIL: Not safe for use on injured or damaged skin, may be contaminated with 1,4-dioxane.

PEG-100 STEARATE: all polyethylene glycols are often contaminated with 1,4-dioxane; suspected endocrine disruptor; linked to cancer in animals; skin and eye irritant.

PETROLATUM (soft paraffin, white petrolatum, petroleum jelly): lung irritant upon inhalation; derived from petroleum; nonbiodegradable environmental toxin.

PHENOL: strong respiratory irritant; toxic by skin contact, causes skin burns; causes kidney damage and cyanosis in humans; causes skin cancer, birth defects, brain and nervous system damage in animals at very low doses; environmental contaminant; banned in Canada, restricted in Japan, permitted in the United States.

PHENYLPHENOL: this fragrance component is a strong human neurotoxin and lung toxicant. It is a possible carcinogen restricted for use in cosmetics. Found in cleansers for sensitive skin.

PHENOLPHTHALEIN: this chemical is a human carcinogen and endocrine disruptor. It is found in styling products and shampoo.

PHENOXYETHANOL: endocrine disruptor and carcinogen in animals; linked to allergic contact uritica and dermatitis.

PLACENTAL EXTRACT: endocrine disruptor containing estradiol and progesterone; banned in Canada.

POLYETHYLENE GLYCOL (PEG): often contaminated with carcinogenic 1,4-dioxane; suspected endocrine disruptor; linked to cancer in animals; skin and eye irritant.

POLYETHYLENE TEREPHTHALATE: causes cancer in animals; not studied for safety in humans.

POLYSORBATE 80: may be contaminated with 1,4-dioxane; suspected endocrine disruptor; linked to cancer in animals; skin and eye irritant.

P-PHENYLENEDIAMINE: linked to bladder and prostate cancer; human neurotoxin; skin and lung irritant; causes liver cancer and birth defects in animals; very strong environmental toxin.

PROPYLENE GLYCOL (PG): can cause eye irritation and conjunctivitis, as well as upper respiratory tract irritation; strong skin irritant.

PROPYLPARABEN: skin and eye irritant; endocrine disruptor linked to breast and ovarian cancer; environmental contaminant.

QUATERNIUM-7, 15, 31, 60: formaldehyde releaser; can cause skin and eye irritation; linked to several cancers (see FORMALDEHYDE).

RESORCINOL (m-hydroquinone, euresol, 1,3-benzenediol): strong skin irritant, linked to adenomas in animals, suspected to trigger skin cancer in humans, environmental toxin.

RETINYL PALMITATE (Vitamin A Palmitate): linked to skin cancer, shows reproductive toxicity, and causes DNA mutations.

SACCHARIN: suspected human carcinogen; causes liver, kidney, and bladder damage in animals, as well as reproductive damage and birth abnormalities.

SELENIUM SULFIDE: used in antidandruff treatment, this chemical is toxic to human nervous system and is a possible human carcinogen limited for use in cosmetics.

SODIUM METHYLPARABEN: endocrine disruptor; caused mild brain damage in animals; skin irritant causing itching, burning, scaling, hives, and blistering of skin; causes depigmentation of skin; banned for use in European Union.

SODIUM MONOFLUOROPHOS-PHATE: nervous system toxin; harmful if swallowed during teeth bleaching; causes convulsions, proteinuria, osteoporosis, and changes in DNA in animals; restricted in Canada.

SODIUM LAURETH SULFATE: skin irritant, water contaminant, may be contaminated with carcinogen 1,4-dioxane.

SODIUM SULFITE: immune system toxicant; eye and skin irritant; emits toxic gas when contacts with acids; dangerous for asthmatics; causes stillbirth, muscle weakness, and brain degeneration in animals.

TALC: even when it contains no asbestos, was proven fibrogenic (causes tissue injury and fibrosis), skin and lung irritation.

TETRASODIUM EDTA: contains formaldehyde; cytotoxic and genotoxic in animals; strong skin and lung irritant in humans; most widespread poison to waterways.

THIMEROSAL (Thiomersal, Merthiolate): contains mercury, which is a strong toxin to skin, nervous and immune system; causes cancer in animals; environmental toxin.

THIOGLYCOLIC ACID: contains mercury, strong human skin irritant; causes itching, burning, scaling, hives, and blistering of skin; lung allergen; restricted in cosmetics; banned in Canada.

TOLUENE (methylbenzene): skin and lung toxicant; accumulates in fat tissue; soil contaminant.

TRICLOSAN: endocrine disruptor, affects thyroid hormone-associated gene .expression, caused fetal death in animals;

strong skin irritant; environmental toxicant

TRIETHANOLAMINE (TEA):
causes lymphoid, kidney, and
renal tumors in animals; may be
contaminated with carcinogen
1,4-dioxane; skin and eye irritant even when used in low
doses.

TRIPHENYL PHOSPHATE: this
nail color ingredient is a human
immune system toxicant and
neurotoxin.

VERBENA *(Lippia citriodora)*:
banned for use in fragrances
based on strong evidence of
human toxicity.

XANTHENE (AKA106, CI
45100): found unsafe for use in
cosmetics in the United States;
caused cancer and various organ
mutations in animals.

ZINOXOL: this odor-reducing
chemical is a strong immune
system suppressant and a known
neurotoxin.

SOURCES

Cosmetic Ingredient Review (CIR); Environmental Protection Agency
(EPA); European Union: Classification & Labelling; Health Canada:
List of Prohibited and Restricted Cosmetic Ingredients; EPA Water
Quality Standards Database; EPA Hazardous Air Pollutants; National
Library of Medicine; CHE Toxicant and Disease Database; Scorecard.
org Toxicity Information; U.S. Association of Occupational and En-
vironmental Clinics; International Agency for Research on Cancer
(IARC).

APPENDIX B

Going to make your own natural beauty products? Here are some suggestions to get you started:

NATURAL INGREDIENTS

Mountain Rose Herbs *(www.mountainroseherbs.com)*
Dried herbs, hydrosols, clays, honey, vitamins, and other ingredients for a beauty enthusiast. One of the oldest and most trusted resources for all things green and wholesome.

Texas Natural Supply *(www.texasnaturalsupply.com)*
Vitamins, clays, antioxidants, ready-blended bases, and natural preservatives for organic and natural skincare, haircare, and makeup products delivered worldwide and with great customer service.

From Nature with Love *(www.fromnaturewithlove.com)*
A wholesale supplier of natural ingredients used in skincare, hair care, aromatherapy, massage, and spa products, as well as herbal preparations, soap, and candle-making materials, and potpourri.

Ingredients to Die For (*www.ingredientstodiefor.com*)
Despite the macabre name, this website sells an astonishing selection of vitamins, pre-blended formulas, and organic and semi-natural base formulas for cosmetic enthusiasts in very small quantities.

Essential Wholesale (*www.essentialwholesale.com*)
Basic ingredients, oils, butters, waxes, vitamins, essential oils, mineral pigments, and other ingredients to make your own natural beauty products and makeup.

FOR MORE INFORMATION
ON HOW TO MAKE SKINCARE, MAKEUP,
BODY CARE, AND SOAPS

Green Beauty Recipes: Easy Homemade Recipes to Make Your Own Organic and Natural Skincare, Hair Care and Body Care Products by Julie Gabriel (Petite Marie Books, 2010)

Organic Body Care Recipes: 175 Homemade Herbal Formulas for Glowing Skin & a Vibrant Self by Stephanie Tourles (Storey Publishing, 2007)

The Complete Book of Essential Oils and Aromatherapy: Over 600 Natural, Non-Toxic and Fragrant Recipes to Create Health—Beauty—a Safe Home Environment by Valerie Ann Worwood (New World Library, 1991)

Smart Soapmaking: The Simple Guide to Making Traditional Handmade Soap Quickly, Safely, and Reliably, or How to Make Luxurious Handcrafted Soaps for Family, Friends, and Yourself by Anne L. Watson (Shepard Publications, 2007)

The Naturally Clean Home: 150 Super-Easy Herbal Formulas for Green Cleaning by Karyn Siegel-Maier (Storey Publishing, LLC, 2008)

Homemade: How to Make Hundreds of Everyday Products Fast, Fresh, and More Naturally by Reader's Digest (Readers Digest, 2008)

Return to Beauty: Old-World Recipes for Great Radiant Skin by Narine Nikogosian (Atria Books, 2009)

Advanced Aromatherapy: The Science of Essential Oil Therapy by Kurt Schnaubelt Ph.D. (Healing Arts Press, 1998)

The Hundred-Year Lie: How to Protect Yourself from the Chemicals that Are Destroying Your Health by Randall Fitzgerald (Plume, 2007)

Not Just a Pretty Face: The Ugly Side of the Beauty Industry by Stacy Malkan (New Society Publishers, 2007)

No More Dirty Looks: The Truth about Your Beauty Products and the Ultimate Guide to Safe and Clean Cosmetics by Siobhan O'Connor and Alexandra Spunt (Da Capo Lifelong Books, 2010)

Slow Death by Rubber Duck: The Secret Danger of Everyday Things by Rick Smith, Bruce Lourie (Counterpoint; Reprint edition, 2011)

Food Additives: A Shopper's Guide to What's Safe & What's Not by Christine Hoza Farlow (KISS For Health Publishing, 2007)

Exposed: The Toxic Chemistry of Everyday Products and What's at Stake for American Power by Mark Schapiro (Chelsea Green Publishing, 2009)

The Body Toxic: How the Hazardous Chemistry of Everyday Things Threatens Our Health and Well-Being by Nena Baker (North Point Press, 2009)

APPENDIX C

Recommended
Natural Beauty Brands

When I was writing *The Green Beauty Guide* in 2007, a similar appendix was a lot easier to write, as there were maybe ten reliably green beauty brands. Today, we are spoilt for choice when we choose to go natural in skincare, and therefore, I would rather suggest a brand than a particular product—there are just too many of them, fortunately, to choose from.

I have handpicked the following brands because their products did not contain synthetic chemicals, petrochemicals, harsh preservatives, or artificial fragrance at the time of writing in April 2012. However, product formulations can change, and a pure product can turn into a "green-washed" one overnight. So always do your homework before purchasing!

100% Pure (100percentpure. com): innovative makeup products tinted with fruit and vegetable pigments as well as natural and organic skincare products—including ice cream-flavored, naturally scented baby washes and shampoos.

A'kin (www.purist.com): pure and organic skincare and hair care products enriched with antioxidants and botanicals from Australia.

Alima Pure (www.alimapure. com): lovely mineral makeup without any nasties.

Alqvimia (www.alqvimia.com): the twenty-five-year-old natural and organic skincare line from Spain specializing in aromatherapeutic body products and fragrances.

Amazon Beauty (www.rahua. com): presents a natural hair care brand Rahua that is free from chemicals and full of Amazonian plant extracts.

Antipodes (www.antipodes nature.com): certified organic skincare featuring organic avocado oil blended with exotic New Zealand plant extracts.

Apples & Pears (www.apples-and-pears.com): lovely lip balms with beeswax made entirely by hand. Ideal for sensitive, dry, or baby lips.

Aromafloria (www.aromafloria. com): specializing in aromatherapeutic products for skin and mind.

Babybearshop (www.baby bearshop.com): stocks lovely baby skincare products that are also good for mommies with sensitive dry skin.

Badger Balm (www.badger-balm.com): is one of the pioneers of the green beauty trade. They make the most effective skin balm and, more recently,

the most luxurious natural anti-aging sunscreen, as well as zinc oxide sun creams for children.

Balm Balm (www.balmbalm. com): started with a simple concept, to offer a multifunctional balm to go on lips, lids, cheeks, and anywhere you like. Today, Balm Balm also added single-note natural fragrances to simplify our lives even more.

Barefoot Botanicals (www. barefootbotanicals.com): is a natural skincare line with scientific edge. The brand name was inspired by the ancient Chinese tradition of barefoot doctors who traveled from village to village, supplying remedies and spreading wisdom.

Brown Earth (www.brownearth. co.uk): supplies unrefined organic shea butter (probably the best body moisturizer on the planet) as well as black soap (great for acne) and essential oil-based bath products.

Dr. Alkaitis (www.alkaitis. com): offers organic cleansers, masks, and moisturizers pre-fermented in the lab to increase skin compatibility.

Dr. Bronner's Magic Soaps (www.drbronner.com): my trusted favorite for years. Their soaps clean skin, hair, body, and dishes without any dryness or acrid smells. In fact, you can use one soap (my choice is Baby Mild Liquid Soap) for head-to-toe cleansing and you won't even need a conditioner or a moisturizer. This brand is a self-appointed natural skincare industry watchdog, so rest assured you are washing or shampooing yourself with the cleanest product possible.

Dr. Hauschka (www.drhauschka. com): one of the pioneers of organic and natural skincare. Their exfoliating cleanser paved way to the whole natural cleansing trend. We love their moisturizers and tinted face oils, while their body oils are simply irresistible.

Fresh Therapies (www.fresh therapies.com): makes one stellar product: EDEN Natural Nail Varnish Remover, which is free from acetone or other dangerous chemicals. Smells delicious and actually helps moisturize your nails.

Ecosoapia (www.ecosoapia. com): the UK's answer to Dr. Bronner's natural liquid soaps, although they are a lot more expensive.

Elysambre (www.elysambre. com): a French organic makeup company that sells their powder foundations and blushes in gorgeous refillable packaging. Turn to them for chic shades of natural nail polishes and runway-worthy organic lip colors.

Faith in Nature (www.faith innaturre.com): a British natural skincare company that makes lovely hair and body care products free from toxins and synthetics and yet at very affordable prices.

Florascent (www.florascent. com): makes gorgeous perfumes that are 100 percent natural and free from phthalates.

Herbfarmacy (www.herb farmacy): a British organic skincare for sensitive skin handmade in Herefordshire on the farm from organically grown herbs.

INIKA (www.inika.com.au): creates luxurious mineral powders and certified organic liquid mineral foundations and concealers based on aloe vera juice and enriched with antioxidants and botanical extracts from Australia.

Intelligent Nutrients (www. intelligentnutrients.com): created by Aveda founder Horst M. Rechelbacher. Head to them for lovely hair products, powerful antiaging products, and (my personal favorite) organic Bug Repellant Serum.

John Masters Organics (www.johnmasters.com): created by a hairstylist who realized the serious health risks posed by inhaling and handling harsh salon chemicals. Now, his toxin-free salons dye hair with clays and natural pigments while organic shampoos and conditioners deliver impressive results and smell naturally fantastic.

Konjac Sponge Company (www.konjacspongecompany.com): nature's answer to the Clarisonic brush: a natural sponge infused with clays and bamboo charcoal to exfoliate and deeply cleanse the skin. I love their baby sponge, which can also be used for mineral makeup application.

L'Artisan Parfumeur (www.artisanparfumeur.com): one of the most unique natural fragrance houses. Turn to them for natural musk scents as well as unmistakably French charming perfume concoctions.

LEAP Organics (www.leaporganics.com): proves that organic body washes do not have to cost the earth to be sumptuous and effective. Certified USDA organic, vegan and cruelty-free skincare is poured in recycled packaging and each sale supports environment-protecting charities.

Madara (www.madara.com): makes lovely skincare hair care products using herbals from the Baltic Sea. They also have a really effective herbal deodorant without aluminum.

Moom (www.moom.com): organic hair removal products combine the ancient art of sugaring with traditional waxing. Moom products are free from synthetics and are delicate enough to use on sensitive skin. For the first time, hair removal products also customized for use by men.

Natural Being (www.naturalbeingskincare.com): a simple, certified organic antiaging line from New Zealand. Its products are entirely based on Manuka honey and Manuka oil.

Nvey Eco (www.nveyeco.com): makes certified organic makeup including brightly colored lipsticks that are just too good to be naturally pigmented (still, they are). I love their foundations enriched with botanical extracts and antioxidants.

Oskia (www.oskia.com): makes potent antiaging, anti-blemish skincare with youth-boosting vitamins, minerals, prebiotics, essential fatty acids, and methyl sulphonyl methane (MSM) for collagen maintenance.

Pai (www.paiskincare.com): a British skincare range which is excellent for sensitive skin or suffering from skin conditions such as eczema, rosacea, urticaria, and contact dermatitis.

Pangea Organics (www. pangea organics.com): an aromatherapeutic collection of face and body products that benefit the mind, body, and planet without any synthetics or petrochemicals, and their packaging is infused with plant seeds so you can put them into soil and grow flowers.

Patyka (www.patyka.com): makes adorable all-natural fragrances and potent antiaging creams, masks, and cleansers.

Petite Marie Organics (www. petitemarieorganics.com): an organic skincare line for oily, acne-prone skin. They also have a new mom-and-baby range, Mamaria, formulated with 100 percent natural, food-grade ingredients and handmade in England.

Primavera (www.primavera. com): makes certified organic essential oils, energizing room sprays, organic floral waters,

aromatherapeutic roll-on treatments, and divine body care products.

Raw Elements (www.raw elementsusa.com): sunscreens are natural sunblocks made with over 70 percent certified organic ingredients, using mineral zinc oxide, and carry the top rating by The Environmental Working Group for safety.

Santaverde (www.santaverde. com): make lovely skincare products which are extra soothing and thus great for sensitive skin. They simply took away the water from their creams and replaced it with organic aloe juice from their farm in Andalusia in Spain. Brilliant!

Suki (www.sukipure.com): features innovative organic skincare products with a strong scientific edge. All their products are made with 100 percent synthetic-free and organic ingredients.

Suncoat (www.suncoatproducts. com): makes truly innovative organic beauty products such as water-based nail polishes and removers, sugar-basedhair styling products, and talc-free makeup.

Tallulah Jane (www.tallulah jane.com): exquisite natural fragrances made from organic and wild-crafted oils infused in certified organic grape alcohol or jojoba oil, then hand-poured in small batches. Naturally free from phthalates or solvents.

UNE (www.unebeauty.com): an organic child of a famous Bourgeois makeup brand from France. Made from entirely natural ingredients, UNE lip, eye, and face makeup products are of excellent quality and shades are very wearable too.

Weleda (www.weleda.com): a true pioneer of green beauty. Founded more than ninety years ago in Germany, Weleda makes gorgeous face and body products as well as homeopathic remedies. Their baby line is one of the few that are not loaded with synthetic scents or alcohol.

Zoya (www.zoya.com): founded by pregnant "nail lady" Zoya Rivkin, who was determined to stop ruining her health by formaldehyde vapors. Result is a professional quality nail polish range free of toluene, formaldehyde, phthalates, and camphor. Zoya polishes come in a zillion of chic, wearable shades and have incredible staying power.

APPENDIX D

Helpful Lists for Your Pocketbook

10 BEST FOODS FOR EMOTIONAL WELL-BEING

1. Greens: kale, chard, mustard greens
2. Oats
3. Pumpkin seeds
4. Dark chocolate
5. Flax and sesame seed oil and butter
6. Brazil nuts
7. Spelt
8. Brown rice
9. Herbs: chives, sage, dill, basil
10. Spinach

10 BEST FOODS FOR BETTER SLEEP

1. Oats
2. Pumpkin and sesame seeds
3. Cherries
4. Shellfish, especially scallops and oysters
5. Almonds

6. Buckwheat
7. Artichokes
8. Turkey
9. Cheese (in moderation)
10. Beans

10 BEST FOODS FOR YOUR SKIN

1. Fatty fish
2. Oats
3. Brussels sprouts, broccoli, and white cabbage
4. Olive oil
5. Cottage cheese or tofu (if vegan)
6. Leafy greens, chard, salad greens
7. Spinach
8. Berries (blueberries, strawberries, blackberries)
9. Green tea
10. Water

10 BEST FOODS FOR HAIR AND NAILS

1. Fish oil
2. Spinach
3. Eggs
4. Leafy green vegetables
5. Brewer's yeast extract
6. Citrus fruits
7. Potatoes
8. Nuts and seeds
9. Red meat (free range or organic)
10. Apricots

THE DIRTY DOZEN:
12 INGREDIENTS TO AVOID IN SKINCARE

1. Parabens (methylparaben, ethylparaben, butyl-paraben and everything -paraben. Also watch out for para-aminobenzoic acid and Phenotip (contains parabens).

2. Artificial fragrances: watch out for words "perfume" and "fragrance." The only safe fragrances in skincare are derived from essential oils, and responsible manufacturers usually note that on the label.

3. Aluminum: abundant in antiperspirants but also found in sunscreens and makeup, where it's used to create matte effect and reduce perspiration.

4. Formaldehyde: usually listed as formaldehyde resin in nail polishes and hairstyling products.

5. Ethoxylated compounds: anything with -eth in the name, for example, sodium laureth sulfate.

6. Propylene glycol: ubiquitous in deodorants, skincare, toothpastes, and baby products.

7. Lanolin: highly irritating and comedogenic sheep wool alcohol.

8. Denatured alcohol: often listed as "SD-alcohol," this ingredient contains traces of acetone and other toxic substances.

9. Synthetic dyes: watch out for letter and number combinations such as D&C Red 2.

10. Toluene: usually found in nail polishes and artificially scented products; often hides under BHT (butyl hydroxy toluene).

11. Paraffinum: yet another harsh emollient derived from crude oil.

12. Mineral oil: this petrochemical clogs pores and accumulates in the body.

FOXY FIVE:
5 MOST BENEFICIAL INGREDIENTS
IN YOUR SKINCARE

1. Sunblocks: titanium dioxide and zinc oxide protect your skin from all types of sun radiation by reflecting sun rays rather than starting a long-term relationship with them deep in your skin.
2. Plant oils: thin oils like jojoba and thistle deliver useful ingredients into your dermis; thicker oils protect from dehydration and keep skin supple.
3. Vitamins: look for vitamins A, C, and E in the ingredient list. Avoid retinyl palmitate, though, as it has been linked to skin cancer.
4. Antioxidants: look for green tea, pomegranate, resveratrol, grape skin extract, quercetin, curcumin, beta-carotene, and lycopene.
5. Seaweed and algae: these marine beauty boosters nourish the skin with microelements, minerals, proteins, and vitamins in a completely bioavailable form.

GROCERY BEAUTY: SHOPPING LIST
OF COMMON BEAUTY INGREDIENTS

Here is a list of food products that make one-step green beauty products instantly in your kitchen:

Avocado: A ready-made remedy for dry skin, split hair ends, and rough cuticles. Just mash and apply.

Baking soda: Makes a great face and body scrub when mixed with olive or any other oil; can also be used as grainy exfoliating filler for your more intricate masks and scrubs; when added to bathwater, softens the skin.

Cocoa: Dilute with water to make a hair rinse for dark hair.

Coffee: The contents of your coffee filter can be used as a body scrub; very strong brewed (cool) coffee is a great hair rinse for dark hair.

Cornstarch: Soothing, tightening, and mildly exfoliating agent for masks and scrubs.

Eggs: Can be massaged into the hair as a nourishing conditioner; egg whites are a traditional face-lifting remedy.

Chamomile tea: Can be used as a toner, hair rinse for blonde hair, and a general purpose calming skin and hair mist.

Green tea: A great all-purpose skin toner, face mask, and scrub filler, eye soother, and a baby skin rinse if your little one suffers from eczema.

Honey: An antibacterial ingredient, a soothing face mask, and a very useful cure for dandruff—just add some honey to your shampoo.

Lemons: The juice makes a gorgeous skin-whitening and hair-lightening treatment; rind can be used to scent the bathwater; oil squeezed from the rind works magic on acne blemishes.

Mayonnaise: Gorgeous moisturizer for face, body, and especially feet.

Milk: Use it to wipe your face after cleansing for

mildly exfoliating effect; add to bathwater to soften the skin; rinse your hair for added volume and to combat dryness.

Milk of magnesia: Very effective mask for acne, sunburns, and eczema.

Oranges: Cut them in half and add to your bathwater along with olive oil.

Vegetable oils: Should be your number one beauty ingredient. Vegetable oils can be added to the face cream, as a massage oil, bath oil, or body/face scrubs. Great skin-friendly oils to explore include grapeseed, rice bran, hemp, castor seed, jojoba, and sesame oils.

Salt: Works great as a face and body exfoliating agent, especially useful for instant manicures. Look for very fine sea salt, which will not damage your skin.

Sugar: Can be used in face and body scrubs.

Oatmeal: make them into scrubs, face masks, bath pouches.

Tomatoes: Revive tired skin and hair to help it look shiny and smooth.

Yogurt: Works really well as an exfoliating face mask and to combat dry, itchy scalp.

ACKNOWLEDGMENTS

I want to thank the outstanding team of people that helped me to conceive, write, revise, and produce this new book.

To all my dear friends, my mother Lilia, my daughter Maria, my best friend Tatiana, and my readers who share my passion for natural beauty and holistic well-being. Your support, your feedback, and your invaluable ideas are precious to me.

I send heartfelt thanks to my editor Crystal Yakacki: Thank you for your faith in me, your direction, your insight in improving my work, and your patience with me.

Also, I thank Stewart Cauley for the stunning cover design.

A special thank you to Dr. Victoria Fleming for explaining the psychological concept (and consequences) of striving to be beautiful at all costs. Another thank you to yoga gurus Devinder Kaur and Paul Smith, for making the quest for truly natural beauty a lot more enjoyable.

A final thank you to everyone at Seven Stories Press for their time and effort; your kindness, your warm attitude, and your support make my job a pure pleasure. You deserve a bit of holistic, kind beauty, and I hope you make good use of my recipes. I feel privileged to create yet another inspiring story for Seven Stories!

ABOUT THE AUTHOR

JULIE GABRIEL is a journalist and holistic nutritionist educated at the Canadian School for Natural Nutrition in Toronto, Canada. During her career as a beauty journalist and editor, she worked for many glossy publications including *Harper's Bazaar, Women's Wear Daily,* and *L'Officiel De La Mode et De La Couture.* During her pregnancy, Julie discovered how toxic common beauty and household products can be and became determined to teach other new moms how to take care of their skin and hair naturally and holistically while avoiding damaging toxic chemicals.

As a practitioner of holistic nutrition and wellness, Julie has great interest in symptomatic nutrition, which is concerned with the effects of vitamins, phytonutrients, antioxidants, and minerals in our food on various health conditions and human health in general.

Since 2008, Julie has been formulating organic beauty products for her own skincare brand Petite Marie Organics (www. petitemarieorganics.com), named after her little daughter, Marie. All skincare products are created by hand using local, organic, and ethically harvested botanicals, clays, and vitamins. Petite Marie Organics skincare range is free from synthetics of any kind.

OTHER BOOKS BY JULIE GABRIEL

The Green Beauty Guide: Your Essential Resource to Organic and Natural Skin Care, Hair Care, Makeup, and Fragrances (HCI, 2008)

    Green Beauty Recipes: Easy Homemade Recipes to Create your Own Organic and Natural Skincare, Hair Care and Body Care Products (Petite Marie; 2010)

    The Acne Diet: Holistic Plan to Achieve Clear, Youthful, Acne-Free Skin with Natural Nutrition, Stress Relief and Organic Skincare (Pure Vitality Books, 2012).

MORE INFORMATION

The Green Beauty Guide (www.thegreenbeautyguide.com)
Petite Marie Organics (www.petitemarieorganics.com)

NOTES

1. Cathy Newman. *The Enigma of Beauty.* http://science.national geographic.com/science/health-and-human-body/human-body/ enigma-beauty. Accessed May 21, 2012.

2. Platek SM, Singh D. *Optimal waist-to-hip ratios in women activate neural reward centers in men.* PLoS One. 2010 Feb 5; 5(2): e9042.

3. Rebecca Penzer, Steven Esser. *Principles of Skin Care: A Guide for Nurses and Health Practitioners.* http://www.ola.tm/downloads/Principles_of_Skin_ Care.pdf: 22–23. Accessed September 7, 2012.

4. Dirmaier J, Steinmann M, Krattenmacher T, Watzke B, Barghaan D, Koch U, Schulz H. *Non-pharmacological treatment of depressive disorders: a review of evidence-based treatment options.* Review of Recent Clinical Trials. 2012 May; 7(2): 141–9.

5. "Few women 'happy with their bodies'," BBC News World Edition, http://news.bbc.co.uk/2/hi/health/2402363.stm. Accessed September 9, 2012.

6. Lam LC, Chau RC, Wong BM, Fung AW, Tam CW, Leung GT, Kwok TC, Leung TY, Ng SP, Chan WM. *A 1-Year Randomized Controlled Trial Comparing Mind Body Exercise (Tai Chi) With Stretching and Toning Exercise on Cognitive Function in Older Chinese Adults at Risk of Cognitive Decline.* Journal of American Medical Directors Association. 2012 May 11. (Published ahead of print, accessed via pubmed.com on May 22, 2012.)

7. McConnell AR, Brown CM, Shoda TM, Stayton LE, Martin CE. *Friends with benefits: on the positive consequences of pet ownership.* Journal of Personal and Social Psychology. 2011 Dec; 101(6): 1239–52.

8. Louisa Peacock. "Stress overtakes cancer as main cause of sickness absence," The Telegraph, http://www.telegraph.co.uk/finance/

jobs/8806473/Stress-overtakes-cancer-as-main-cause-of-sickness-absence.html. Accessed September 7, 2012.

9. Platek SM, Singh D. Ignacchiti MD, Sesti-Costa R, Marchi LF, Chedraoui-Silva S, Mantovani B. *Effect of academic psychological stress in post-graduate students: the modulatory role of cortisol on superoxide release by neutrophils.* Stress. 2011; 14(3): 290–300.

10. Sánchez-Villegas A, Delgado-Rodríguez M, Alonso A, Schlatter J, Lahortiga F, Serra Majem L, Martínez-González MA. *Association of the Mediterranean dietary pattern with the incidence of depression: the Seguimiento Universidad de Navarra/University of Navarra follow-up (SUN) cohort.* Archives of General Psychiatry. 2009 Oct; 66(10): 1090–8.

11. Demetriou CA, Hadjisavvas A, Loizidou MA, Loucaides G, Neophytou I, Sieri S, Kakouri E, Middleton N, Vineis P, Kyriacou K. *The Mediterranean dietary pattern and breast cancer risk in Greek–Cypriot women: A case-control study.* BMC Cancer. 2012 Mar 23; 12(1): 113.

12. Deyama T, Nishibe S, Nakazawa Y. *Constituents and pharmacological effects of Eucommia and Siberian ginseng.* Acta Pharmacologica Sinica. 2001 Dec; 22(12): 1057–70.

13. Edwards D, Heufelder A, Zimmermann A. *Therapeutic Effects and Safety of Rhodiola rosea Extract WS® 1375 in Subjects with Life-stress Symptoms—Results of an Open-label Study.* Phytotherapy Research. 2012 Jan 6. doi: 10.1002/ptr.3712.

14. Bhattacharya SK, Muruganandam AV. *Adaptogenic activity of Withania somnifera: an experimental study using a rat model of chronic stress.* Pharmacology, Biochemistry and Behaviour. 2003 Jun; 75(3): 547–55.

15. Rosenzweig S, Greeson JM, Reibel DK, et al. *Mindfulness-based stress reduction for chronic pain conditions: variation in treatment outcomes and role of home meditation practice.* Journal of Psychosomatic Research 2010; 68: 29–36.

16. Astin JA. Stress reduction through mindfulness meditation. *Effects psychological symptomatology, sense control, spiritual experiences.* Psychotherapy and Psychosomatics 1997; 66: 97–106.

17. Kingston J, Chadwick P, Meron D, et al. *A pilot randomized control trial investigating the effect of mindfulness practice on pain tolerance, psychological well-being, and physiological activity.* Journal of Psychosomatic Research 2007; 62: 297–300.

18. Grossman P, Tiefenthaler-Gilmer U, Raysz A, et al. *Mindfulness*

training as an intervention for fibromyalgia: evidence of postintervention and 3-year follow-up benefits in well-being. Psychotherapy and Psychosomatics 2007; 76: 226–33.

19. Kristeller JL, Hallett CB. *An exploratory study of a meditation-based intervention for binge eating disorder.* Journal of Health Psychology, 1999; 4: 357–63

20. Kabat-Zinn J, Wheeler E, Light T, et al. *Influence of a mindfulness meditation-based stress reduction intervention on rates of skin clearing in patients with moderate to severe psoriasis undergoing phototherapy (UVB) and photochemotherapy (PUVA).* Psychosomatic Medicine 1998; 60: 625–32.

21. Rosenzweig S, Reibel DK, Greeson JM, et al. *Mindfulness-based stress reduction is associated with improved glycemic control in type 2 diabetes mellitus: a pilot study.* Alternative Therapies in Health and Medicine 2007; 13: 36–8.

22. Shumate M. *Transcendental meditation: its application to the stress of life.* NLN Publications. 1977; (16–1674): 63–9.

23. Yadav RK, Ray RB, Vempati R, Bijlani RL. *Effect of a comprehensive yoga-based lifestyle modification program on lipid peroxidation.* Indian Journal of Physiology and Pharmacology. 2005 Jul-Sep; 49(3): 358–62.

24. Brand S, Holsboer-Trachsler E, Naranjo JR, Schmidt S. *Influence of mindfulness practice on cortisol and sleep in long-term and short-term meditators.* Neuropsychobiology 2012; 65(3): 109–18.

25. Liou CH, Hsieh CW, Hsieh CH, Chen DY, Wang CH, Chen JH, Lee SC. *Detection of nighttime melatonin level in Chinese Original Quiet Sitting.* Journal of the Formosan Medical Association. 2010 Oct; 109(10): 694–701.

26. Martarelli D, Cocchioni M, Scuri S, Pompei P. *Diaphragmatic Breathing Reduces Exercise-induced Oxidative Stress.* Evidence Based Complementary and Alternative Medicine. 2009 Oct 29.

27. Liou CH, Hsieh CW, Hsieh CH, Chen DY, Wang CH, Chen JH, Lee SC. *Detection of night-time melatonin level in Chinese Original Quiet Sitting.* Journal of Formosan Medical Association. 2010 Oct; 109(10): 694–701.

28. Nidhi R, Padmalatha V, Nagarathna R, Ram A. *Effect of a yoga program on glucose metabolism and blood lipid levels in adolescent girls with polycystic ovary syndrome.* Interational Journal of Gynaecology and Obstetrics. 2012 Apr 14.

29. Sinha S, Singh SN, Monga YP, Ray US. *Improvement of glutathione and total antioxidant status with yoga.* Journal of Alternative and Complementary Medicine 2007 Dec; 13(10): 1085–90.

30. Carlson LE, Speca M, Patel KD, Goodey E. *Mindfulness-based stress reduction in relation to quality of life, mood, symptoms of stress and levels of cortisol, dehydroepiandrosterone sulfate (DHEAS) and melatonin in breast and prostate cancer outpatients.* Psychoneuroendocrinology. 2004 May; 29(4): 448–74.

31. Sadlier M, Stephens SD, Kennedy V. *Tinnitus rehabilitation: a mindfulness meditation cognitive behavioural therapy approach.* Journal of Laryngology and Otolaryngology 2008 Jan; 122(1): 31–7.

32. Goldstein CM, Josephson R, Xie S, Hughes JW. *Current perspectives on the use of meditation to reduce blood pressure.* International Journal of Hypertension 2012; 2012: 5783–97.

33. Moliver N, Mika E, Chartrand M, Burrus S, Haussmann R, Khalsa S. *Increased Hatha yoga experience predicts lower body mass index and reduced medication use in women over 45 years.* International Journal of Yoga 2011 Jul; 4(2): 77–86.

34. Garabadu D, Shah A, Ahmad A, Joshi VB, Saxena B, Palit G, Krishnamurthy S. *Eugenol as an antistress agent: modulation of hypothalamic-pituitary-adrenal axis and brain monoaminergic systems in a rat model of stress.* Stress 2011 Mar; 14(2): 145–55.

35. Axelsson J, Sundelin T, Ingre M, Van Someren EJ, Olsson A, Lekander M., *Beauty sleep: experimental study on the perceived health and attractiveness of sleep deprived people.* BMJ 2010 Dec 14; 341:c6614. doi: 10.1136/bmj.c6614.

36. Stevens RG, Rea MS. *Light in the built environment: potential role of circadian disruption in endocrine disruption and breast cancer.* Cancer Causes and Control: CCC. 2001 Apr; 12(3): 279–87.

37. Spiegel K, Leproult R, Van Cauter E. *Impact of Sleep Debt on Metabolic and Endocrine Function.* Lancet 1999 (354):1435-1439.

38. Solarz DE, Mullington JM, Meier-Ewert HK. *Sleep, inflammation and cardiovascular disease.* Frontiers in Bioscience (Elite Edition). 2012 Jun 1; 4: 2490–501.

39. Fang J, Wheaton AG, Keenan NL, Greenlund KJ, Perry GS, Croft JB. *Association of sleep duration and hypertension among US adults varies by age and sex.* American Journal of Hypertension. 2012 Mar; 25(3): 335–41. doi: 10.1038/ajh.2011.201.

40. Martella D, Plaza V, Estévez AF, Castillo A, Fuentes LJ. *Minimizing sleep deprivation effects in healthy adults by differential outcomes.* Acta Psychologica. 2012 Mar; 139(3): 391–6.

41. Sagaspe P, Sanchez-Ortuno M, Charles A, Taillard J, Valtat C, Bioulac B, Philip P. *Effects of sleep deprivation on Color-Word, Emotional, and Specific Stroop interference and on self-reported anxiety.* Brain and Cognition. 2006 Feb; 60(1): 76–87. Epub 2005 Nov 28.

42. Kamphuis J, Meerlo P, Koolhaas JM, Lancel M. *Poor sleep as a potential causal factor in aggression and violence.* Sleep Medicine. 2012 Apr; 13(4): 327–34.

43. von Ruesten A, Weikert C, Fietze I, Boeing H. *Association of Sleep Duration with Chronic Diseases in the European Prospective Investigation into Cancer and Nutrition (EPIC)-Potsdam Study.* PLoS One. 2012; 7(1): e30972.

44. Zizi F, Pandey A, Murrray-Bachmann R, Vincent M, McFarlane S, Ogedegbe G, Jean-Louis G. *Race/Ethnicity, sleep duration, and diabetes mellitus: analysis of the national health interview survey.* The American Journal of Medicine. 2012 Feb; 125(2): 162–7.

45. Costa G. *Shift work and breast cancer.* (Article in Italian) Giornale Italiano di Medicina del Lavoro ed Ergonomia. 2010 Oct-Dec; 32(4): 454–7.

46. Rosales-Corral SA, Acuña-Castroviejo D, Coto-Montes A, Boga JA, Manchester LC, Fuentes-Broto L, Korkmaz A, Ma S, Tan DX, Reiter RJ. *Alzheimer's disease: pathological mechanisms and the beneficial role of melatonin.* Journal of Pineal Research. 2012 Mar; 52(2): 167–202. doi: 10.1111/j.1600-079X.2011.00937.x. E

47. Willis GL, Moore C, Armstrong SM. *A historical justification for and retrospective analysis of the systematic application of light therapy in Parkinson's disease.* Reviews in Neurosciences. 2012 Mar 1; 23(2): 199–226. doi: 10.1515/revneuro-2011-0072.

48. Crooke A, Colligris B, Pintor J. *Update in glaucoma medicinal chemistry: emerging evidence for the importance of melatonin analogues.* Current Medicinal Chemistry. 2012 Jul 1; 19(21): 3508–22.

49. Khaleghipour S, Masjedi M, Ahade H, Enayate M, Pasha G, Nadery F, Ahmadzade G. *Morning and nocturnal serum melatonin rhythm levels in patients with major depressive disorder: an analytical cross-sectional study.* Sao Paulo Medical Journal. 2012; 130(3): 167–72.

50. Suba Z. *Light deficiency confers breast cancer risk by endocrine disorders.* Recent Patients on Anticancer Drug Discovery. 2012 Sep 1; 7(3): 337–44.

51. Sigurdardottir LG, Valdimarsdottir UA, Fall K, Rider JR, Lockley SW, Schernhammer E, Mucci LA. *Circadian disruption, sleep loss, and prostate cancer risk: a systematic review of epidemiologic studies.* Cancer Epidemiology, Biomarkers and Prevention. 2012 Jul; 21(7): 1002–11.

52. Carbajo-Pescador S, García-Palomo A, Martín-Renedo J, Piva M, González-Gallego J, Mauriz JL. *Melatonin modulation of intracellular signaling pathways in hepatocarcinoma HepG2 cell line: role of the MT1 receptor.* Journal of Pineal Research. 2011 Nov; 51(4): 463–71. doi: 10.1111/j.1600-079X.2011.00910.x.

53. Poole EM, Schernhammer ES, Tworoger SS. *Rotating night shift work and risk of ovarian cancer.* Cancer Epidemiology, Biomarkers and Prevention. 2011 May; 20(5): 934–8.

54. Motilva V, García-Mauriño S, Talero E, Illanes M. *New paradigms in chronic intestinal inflammation and colon cancer: role of melatonin.* Journal of Pineal Research. 2011 Aug;5 1(1): 44–60. doi: 10.1111/j.1600-079X.2011.00915.x.

55. Desotelle JA, Wilking MJ, Ahmad N. *The circadian control of skin and cutaneous photodamage(†).* Photochem Photobiol. 2012 Sep; 88(5): 1037–47. doi: 10.1111/j.1751-1097.2012.01099.x

56. Srinivasan V, Pandi-Perumal SR, Cardinali DP, Poeggeler B, Hardeland R. *Melatonin in Alzheimer's disease and other neurodegenerative disorders.* Behavior and Brain Functioning. 2006 May 4; 2: 15.

57. Figueiro MG, Rea MS. *Preliminary evidence that light through the eyelids can suppress melatonin and phase shift dim light melatonin onset.* BMC Research Notes. 2012 May 7; 5(1): 221.

58. Li Q, Zheng T, Holford TR, Boyle P, Zhang Y, Dai M. *Light at night and breast cancer risk: results from a population-based case-control study in Connecticut, USA.* Cancer Causes & Controls. 2010 Dec; 21(12): 2281–5.

59. West KE, Jablonski MR, Warfield B, Cecil KS, James M, Ayers MA, Maida J, Bowen C, Sliney DH, Rollag MD, Hanifin JP, Brainard GC. *Blue light from light-emitting diodes elicits a dose-dependent suppression of melatonin in humans.* The Journal of Applied Physiology. 2011 Mar; 110(3): 619–26.

60. Kvaskoff M, Weinstein P. *Are some melanomas caused by artificial light?* Medical Hypotheses. 2010 Sep; 75(3): 305–11.

61. Peplonska B, Bukowska A, Sobala W, Reszka E, Gromadzinska J, Wasowicz W, Lie JA, Kjuus H, Ursin G. *Rotating night shift work and mammographic density.* Cancer Epidemiology, Biomarkers and Prevention. 2012 Jul; 21(7): 1028–37.

62. Kloog I, Portnov BA, Rennert HS, Haim A. *Does the modern urbanized sleeping habitat pose a breast cancer risk?* Chronobiology International. 2011 Feb; 28(1): 76–80.

63. Reiter RJ, Tan DX, Korkmaz A, Erren TC, Piekarski C, Tamura H, Manchester LC. *Light at night, chronodisruption, melatonin suppression, and cancer risk: a review.* Critical Reviews in Oncogenesis. 2007 Dec; 13(4): 303–28.

64. Marina Kvaskoff and Philip Weinstein, *Are Some Melanomas Caused by Artificial Light?* Medical Hypothesis 75 (3): 305-311.

65. Patel SR, Malhotra A, White DP, Gottlieb DJ, Hu FB. *Association between reduced sleep and weight gain in women.* American Journal of Epidemiology. 2006 Nov 15; 164(10): 947–54.

66. Kuo LE, Czarnecka M, Kitlinska JB, Tilan JU, Kvetnanský R, Zukowska Z. *Chronic stress, combined with a high-fat/high-sugar diet, shifts sympathetic signaling toward neuropeptide Y and leads to obesity and the metabolic syndrome.* Annals of the New York Academy of Sciences. 2008 Dec; 1148: 232–7.

67. Nassa M, Anand P, Jain A, Chhabra A, Jaiswal A, Malhotra U, Rani V. *Analysis of human collagen sequences.* Bioinformation. 2012; 8(1): 26–33.

68. Liang J, Pei X, Zhang Z, Wang N, Wang J, Li Y. *The protective effects of long-term oral administration of marine collagen hydrolysate from chum salmon on collagen matrix homeostasis in the chronological aged skin of Sprague-Dawley male rats.* Journal of Food Sciences. 2010 Oct; 75(8): H230–8. doi: 10.1111/j.1750-3841.2010.01782.x.

69. Demetriou CA, Hadjisavvas A, Loizidou MA, Loucaides G, Neophytou I, Sieri S, Kakouri E, Middleton N, Vineis P, Kyriacou K. *The Mediterranean dietary pattern and breast cancer risk in Greek-Cypriot women: a case-control study.* BMC Cancer. 2012 Mar 23; 12: 113.

70. Danby FW. *Nutrition and aging skin: sugar and glycation. Clinics in Dermatology.* 2010 Jul-Aug; 28(4): 409–11.

71. Li Q, Holford TR, Zhang Y, Boyle P, Mayne ST, Dai M, Zheng T. *Dietary fiber intake and risk of breast cancer by menopausal and estrogen receptor status.* European Journal of Nutrition. 2012 Feb 16. Published on Pubmed.com ahead of print. http://www.ncbi.nlm.nih.gov/pubmed/22350922. Accessed September 9, 2012.

72. Wise LA, Radin RG, Palmer JR, Kumanyika SK, Boggs DA, Rosenberg L. *Intake of fruit, vegetables, and carotenoids in relation to risk of uterine leiomyomata.* American Journal of Clinical Nutrition. 2011 Dec; 94(6): 1620–31.

73. Khan N, Afaq F, Mukhtar H. *Cancer chemoprevention through dietary antioxidants: progress and promise.* Antioxidants & Redox Signaling. 2008 Mar; 10(3): 475–510.

74. Ellis LZ, Liu W, Luo Y, Okamoto M, Qu D, Dunn JH, Fujita M. *Green tea polyphenol epigallocatechin-3-gallate suppresses melanoma growth by inhibiting inflammasome and IL-1ß secretion.* Biochemical and Biophysical Research Communications. 2011 Oct 28; 414(3): 551–6.

75. Chung JH, Han JH, Hwang EJ, Seo JY, Cho KH, Kim KH, Youn JI, Eun HC. *Dual mechanisms of green tea extract (EGCG)-induced cell survival in human epidermal keratinocytes.* FASEB Journal. 2003 Oct; 17(13): 1913–5.

76. Vaid M, Katiyar SK. *Molecular mechanisms of inhibition of photocarcinogenesis by silymarin, a phytochemical from milk thistle (Silybum marianum L. Gaertn.)* International Journal of Oncology. 10 May; 36(5): 1053–60.

77. Fazekas Z, Gao D, Saladi RN, Lu Y, Lebwohl M, Wei H. *Protective effects of lycopene against ultraviolet B-induced photodamage.* Nutrition and Cancer. 2003; 47(2): 181–7.

78. Wiemels J. *Perspectives on the causes of childhood leukemia.* Chemico-Biological Interactions. 2012 Apr 5; 196(3): 59–67.

79. Celik-Ozenci C, Tasatargil A, Tekcan M, Sati L, Gungor E, Isbir M, Usta MF, Akar ME, Erler F. *Effect of abamectin exposure on semen parameters indicative of reduced sperm maturity: a study on farmworkers in Antalya (Turkey).* Andrologia. 2012 Apr 24. doi: 10.1111/j.1439-0272.2012.01297.x.

80. Mariussen E. *Neurotoxic effects of perfluoroalkylated compounds: mechanisms of action and environmental relevance.* Archives of Toxicology. 2012 Sep; 86(9): 1349–67.

81. Coskun R, Gundogan K, Tanriverdi F, Guven M, Sungur M.

Effects of endosulfan intoxication on pituitary functions. Clinical Toxicology. 2012 Jun; 50(5): 441–3.

82. Chighizola C, Meroni PL. *The role of environmental estrogens and autoimmunity.* Autoimmunity Reviews. 2012 May;11(6–7):A493–501.

83. de Cock M, Maas YG, van de Bor M. *Does perinatal exposure to endocrine disruptors induce autism spectrum and attention deficit hyperactivity disorders? Review.* Acta Paediatrica. 2012 Aug; 101(8): 811–8. doi: 10.1111/j.1651-2227.2012.02693.x.

84. Reuters Health, "Underactive Thyroid Linked to Pesticide Exposure," Reuters, February 12, 2010, accessed March 7, 2013, http://www.reuters.com/article/2010/02/12/us-underactive-thyroid-idUSTRE61B54U20100212.

85. Zapata PJ, Tucker GA, Valero D, Serrano M. *Quality parameters and antioxidant properties in organic and conventionally grown broccoli after pre-storage hot water treatment.* Journal of the Science of Food and Agriculture. 2012 Aug 30. doi: 10.1002/jsfa.5865. Published online ahead of print. http://www.ncbi.nlm.nih.gov/pubmed/22936597 Accessed September 9, 2012.

86. Koh E, Charoenprasert S, Mitchell AE. *Effect of organic and conventional cropping systems on ascorbic acid, vitamin C, flavonoids, nitrate, and oxalate in 27 varieties of spinach (Spinacia oleracea L.).* Journal of Agricultural and Food Chemistry. 2012 Mar 28; 60(12): 3144–50.

87. Norberg-Hodge H, Merrifield T, Gorelick S. *Bringing the Food Economy Home: Local Alternatives to Global Agribusiness.* Bloomfield, CT: Kumarian Press, Inc., 2002.

88. Bos JD, Meinardi MM. The 500 Dalton rule for the skin penetration of chemical compounds and drugs. Experimental Dermatology. 2000 Jun; 9(3): 165–9.

89. Sitruk-Ware R. *Transdermal delivery of steroids.* Contraception. 1989 Jan; 39(1): 1–20.

90. Demierre AL, Peter R, Oberli A, Bourqui-Pittet M. Dermal penetration of bisphenol A in human skin contributes marginally to total exposure. Toxicology Letters. 2012 Sep 18; 213(3): 305–8.

91. Pedersen S, Marra F, Nicoli S, Santi P. In vitro skin permeation and retention of parabens from cosmetic formulations. International Journal of Cosmetic Science. 2007 Oct; 29(5): 361–7.

92. "Toxicology and Our Daily Lives," in *Toxlearn Module 1: Introduction to*

Toxicology and Dose-Response. http://toxlearn.nlm.nih.gov/Toxicology/txoioioi/txoioioi.pdf. Accessed September 10, 2012.

93. Crinnion WJ. *Toxic effects of the easily avoidable phthalates and parabens.* Altern Med Rev. 2010 Sep; 15(3): 190–6.

94. Barr L, Metaxas G, Harbach CA, Savoy LA, Darbre PD. *Measurement of paraben concentrations in human breast tissue at serial locations across the breast from axilla to sternum.* Journal of Applied Toxicology. 2012 Mar;32(3):219–32. doi: 10.1002/jat.1786.

95. Pugazhendhi D, Pope GS, Darbre PD. *Oestrogenic activity of p-hydroxybenzoic acid (common metabolite of paraben esters) and methylparaben in human breast cancer cell lines.* Journal of Applied Toxicology. 2005 Jul-Aug; 25(4): 301–9.

96. Zhang L, Freeman LE, Nakamura J, Hecht SS, Vandenberg JJ, Smith MT, Sonawane BR. Formaldehyde and leukemia: epidemiology, potential mechanisms, and implications for risk assessment. Environmental and Molecular Mutagenicity. 2010 Apr; 51(3): 181–91.

97. National Toxicology Program. *Final Report on Carcinogens Background Document for Formaldehyde.* Report on Carcinogens Background Document for Formaldehyde. 2010 Jan; (10–5981): i-512.

98. National Toxicology Program. *Final Report on Carcinogens Background Document for Formaldehyde.* Report on Carcinogens Background Document. 2010 Jan; (10–5981): i-512.

99. Huang LP, Lee CC, Hsu PC, Shih TS. *The association between semen quality in workers and the concentration of di(2-ethylhexyl) phthalate in polyvinyl chloride pellet plant air.* Fertility and Sterility. 2011 Jul; 96(1): 90–4.

100. Hsieh TH, Tsai CF, Hsu CY, Kuo PL, Lee JN, Chai CY, Hou MF, Chang CC, Long CY, Ko YC, Tsai EM. *Phthalates Stimulate the Epithelial to Mesenchymal Transition Through an HDAC6-Dependent Mechanism in Human Breast Epithelial Stem Cells.* Toxicological Sciences. 2012 Aug; 128(2): 365–76.

101. Jurewicz J, Hanke W. *Exposure to phthalates: reproductive outcome and children health. A review of epidemiological studies.* International Journal of Occupational Medicine and Environmental Health. 2011 Jun; 24 (2): 115–41.

102. BalabaniÐ D, Rupnik M, KlemenÐiÐ AK. *Negative impact of endocrine-disrupting compounds on human reproductive health.* Reproduction and Fertility Developments. 2011; 23(3): 403–16.

103. Yen TH, Lin-Tan DT, Lin JL. *Food safety involving ingestion of foods and*

beverages prepared with phthalate-plasticizer-containing clouding agents. Journal of Formosan Medical Association. 2011 Nov; 110(11): 671–84.

104. Kim BN, Cho SC, Kim Y, Shin MS, Yoo HJ, Kim JW, Yang YH, Kim HW, Bhang SY, Hong YC. Phthalates exposure and attention-deficit/hyperactivity disorder in school-age children. Biological Psychiatry. 2009 Nov 15; 66(10): 958–63.

105. Jurewicz J, Hanke W. Exposure to phthalates: reproductive outcome and children health. A review of epidemiological studies. International Journal of Occupational Medicine and Environmental Health. 2011 Jun; 24(2): 115–41.

106. Kolarik B, Naydenov K, Larsson M, Bornehag CG, Sundell J. The association between phthalates in dust and allergic diseases among Bulgarian children. Environmental Health Perspectives. 2008 Jan; 116(1): 98–103.

107. Bornehag CG, Sundell J, Weschler CJ, Sigsgaard T, Lundgren B, Hasselgren M, Hägerhed-Engman L. The association between asthma and allergic symptoms in children and phthalates in house dust: a nested case-control study. Environmental Health Perspectives. 2004 Oct;112(14):1393–7.

108. Bornehag CG, Sundell J, Weschler CJ, Sigsgaard T, Lundgren B, Hasselgren M, Hägerhed-Engman L. The association between asthma and allergic symptoms in children and phthalates in house dust: a nested case-control study. Environmental Health Perspectives. 2004 Oct; 112(14): 1393–7.

109. Jurewicz J, Hanke W. Exposure to phthalates: reproductive outcome and children health. A review of epidemiological studies. International Journal of Occupational Medicine and Environmental Health. 2011 Jun; 24(2): 115–41.

110. Thayer KA, Heindel JJ, Bucher JR, Gallo MA. Role of environmental chemicals in diabetes and obesity: a National Toxicology Program workshop review. Environmental Health Perspectives. 2012 Jun; 120(6): 779–89.

111. Thayer KA, Heindel JJ, Bucher JR, Gallo MA. Role of environmental chemicals in diabetes and obesity: a National Toxicology Program workshop review. Environmental Health Perspectives. 2012 Jun; 120(6): 779–89.

112. Romero-Franco M, Hernández-Ramírez RU, Calafat AM, Cebrián ME, Needham LL, Teitelbaum S, Wolff MS, López-Carrillo L. Personal care product use and urinary levels of phthalate metabolites in Mexican women. Environment International. 2011 Jul; 37(5): 867–71.

113. Shcherbatykh I, Carpenter DO. The role of metals in the etiology of Alzheimer's disease. Journal of Alzheimer's Disease. 2007 May;11(2):191–205.

114. Darbre PD. *Aluminum, antiperspirants and breast cancer.* Journal of Inorganic Biochemistry. 2005 Sep; 99(9): 1912–9.

115. Black RE, Hurley FJ, Havery DC. *Occurrence of 1,4-dioxane in cosmetic raw materials and finished cosmetic products.* Journal of AOAC International. 2001 May-Jun; 84(3): 666–70.

116. Al Jasser M, Mebuke N, de Gannes GC. *Propylene glycol: an often unrecognized cause of allergic contact dermatitis in patients using topical corticosteroids.* Skin Therapy Letter. 2011 May; 16(5): 5–7.

117. Olumide YM, Akinkugbe AO, Altraide D, Mohammed T, Ahamefule N, Ayanlowo S, Onyekonwu C, Essen N. *Complications of chronic use of skin lightening cosmetics.* International Journal of Dermatology. 2008 Apr; 47(4): 344–53.

118. Andersen FA, Bergfeld WF, Belsito DV, Hill RA, Klaassen CD, Liebler DC, Marks JG Jr, Shank RC, Slaga TJ, Snyder PW. *Final amended safety assessment of hydroquinone as used in cosmetics.* International Journal of Toxicology. 2010 Nov-Dec; 29(6 Suppl): 274S-87.

119. Carcinogenicity Assessment Committee. *Hydroquinone (OTC monographed ingredient)* 1996 December 4.

120. Vincent M, Chemarin C. *Health impact of indoor mineral particle pollution.* Revue des Maladies Respiratoires. 2011 Apr; 28(4): 496–502.

121. http://www.fda.gov/ohrms/dockets/dockets/78n0065/78n-0065-mm00003-vol4.pdf. Accessed February 24, 2012.

122. Langseth H, Hankinson SE, Siemiatycki J, Weiderpass E. *Perineal use of talc and risk of ovarian cancer.* Journal of Epidemiology and Community Health. 2008 Apr; 62(4): 358–60.

123. Borzelleca JF, Hogan GK. *Chronic toxicity/carcinogenicity study of FD & C Blue No. 2 in mice.* Food and Chemical Toxicology. 1985 Aug;2 3(8): 719–22.

124. Ganesan L, Margolles-Clark E, Song Y, Buchwald, P. *The food colorant erythrosine is a promiscuous protein-protein interaction inhibitor.* Biochemical Pharmacology. 2011 Mar 15; 81(6): 810–8.

125. Faurschou A, Beyer DM, Schmedes A, Bogh MK, Philipsen PA, Wulf HC. *The relation between sunscreen layer thickness and vitamin D production after ultraviolet B exposure: a randomized clinical trial.* British Journal of Dermatology. 2012 Aug; 167(2): 391–5. doi: 10.1111/j.1365-2133.2012.11004.x.

126. Rizwan M, Rodriguez-Blanco I, Harbottle A, Birch-Machin MA, Watson RE, Rhodes LE. *Tomato paste rich in lycopene protects against cutaneous photodamage in humans in vivo: a randomized controlled trial.* British Journal of Dermatology. 2011 Jan; 164(1): 154–62. doi: 10.1111/j.1365-2133.2010.10057.x.

127. Samson N, Fink B, Matts PJ. *Visible skin condition and perception of human facial appearance.* International Journal of Cosmetic Science. 2010 Jun; 32(3): 167–84.

128. Nohynek GJ, Dufour EK. *Nano-sized cosmetic formulations or solid nanoparticles in sunscreens: A risk to human health?* Archives of Toxicology. March 31, 2012.

129. Preussmann R, Ivankovic S. *Absence of carcinogenic activity in BD rats after oral administration of high doses of bismuth oxychloride.* Food and Cosmetics Toxicology. 1975 Oct; 13(5): 543–4.

130. "Bismuth oxychloride," The Carcinogenic Potency Project. , http://potency.berkeley.edu/chempages/BISMUTH%20 OXYCHLORIDE.html. Accessed September 10, 2012.

131. Gamal EM, Aly EM, Mahmoud SS, Talaat MS, Sallam AS. *FTIR assessment of the effect of Ginkgo biloba leave extract (EGb 761) on mammalian retina.* Cellular Biochemistry and Biophysics. 2011 Sep; 61(1): 169–77.

132. Hsu NY, Lee CC, Wang JY, Li YC, Chang HW, Chen CY, Bornehag CG, Wu PC, Sundell J, Su HJ. *Predicted risk of childhood allergy, asthma, and reported symptoms using measured phthalate exposure in dust and urine.* Indoor Air. 2012 Jun; 22(3): 186–99. doi: 10.1111/j.1600-0668.2011.00753.x.

133. Tsai MJ, Kuo PL, Ko YC. *The association between phthalate exposure and asthma.* Kaohsiung Journal of Medical Science. 2012 Jul; 28(7 Suppl): S28–36.

134. Main KM, Skakkebaek NE, Toppari J. *Cryptorchidism as part of the testicular dysgenesis syndrome: the environmental connection.* Endocrine Development. 2009; 14: 167–73.

135. Roberts JW, Wallace LA, Camann DE, Dickey P, Gilbert SG, Lewis RG, Takaro TK. *Monitoring and reducing exposure of infants to pollutants in house dust.* Reviews of Environmental Contamination and Toxicology. 2009;201:1–39.

136. Tang-Péronard JL, Andersen HR, Jensen TK, Heitmann BL.

Endocrine-disrupting chemicals and obesity development in humans: a review. Obesity Reviews. 2011 Aug; 12(8): 622–36. doi: 10.1111/j.1467-789X.2011.00871.x.

137. Takeuchi S, Iida M, Kobayashi S, Jin K, Matsuda T, Kojima H. *Differential effects of phthalate esters on transcriptional activities via human estrogen receptors alpha and beta, and androgen receptor.* Toxicology. 2005 Jun 1; 210(2–3): 223–33.

138. Victoria Sherrow, *Encyclopedia of Hair: A Cultural History* (New York: Greenwood Publishing Group, 2006), 159–160.

139. Gatherwright J, Liu MT, Gliniak C, Totonchi A, Guyuron B. *The Contribution of Endogenous and Exogenous Factors to Female Alopecia: A Study of Identical Twins.* Plastic and Reconstructive Surgery. August 8, 2012. Published electronically ahead of print . http://www.ncbi.nlm.nih.gov/pubmed/22878477. Accessed September 11, 2012.